CW01663709

SOCIAL AND CULTURAL PERSPECTIVES ON HEALTH, TECHNOLOGY AND MEDICINE: OLD CONCEPTS, NEW PROBLEMS

'This groundbreaking collection puts anthropology and sociology in reflective dialogue with recent developments in science and technology to show how core concepts in both disciplines serve to animate and are themselves reanimated by a diverse range of medical technologies and problems. It provides invaluable theoretical and methodological reflections and resources for situating these disciplines as vital "critical interlocutors" at the centre of contemporary developments in science, medicine and society.'

Sahra Gibbon, University College London, UK

'A truly collaborative text that consistently makes the compelling case that anthropology and sociology are imperative to the production and deconstruction of science, medicine and technology. As bio-medicalization escalates at warp speed and technological innovation is infused in both extraordinary and mundane social life, the authors' sage resurrection of classic concepts advances the integral role of social sciences in critical thinking and daily life.'

Lisa Jean Moore, Purchase College, State University of New York, USA

Developments in health, science and technology have long provided fertile analytical ground for social science disciplines. This book focuses on the critical and enduring importance of core concepts in anthropology and sociology for interrogating and keeping pace with developments in the life sciences. The authors consider how transformations in medical and scientific knowledge serve to reanimate older controversies, giving new life to debates about relations between society, culture, knowledge and individuals. They reflect on the particular legacies and ongoing relevance of concepts such as 'culture', 'society', 'magic', 'production', 'kinship', 'exchange' and 'the body'. The chapters draw on the work of key historical and contemporary figures across the social sciences and include a range of illustrative case studies to explore topics such as transplant medicine, genetic counselling, cancer therapy, reproductive health and addiction. Of particular interest to students and scholars of anthropology, sociology and science and technology studies, this volume will also be a valuable resource for those working in the fields of health and medicine.

Ciara Kierans is a Senior Lecturer in Anthropology in the Department of Public Health and Policy at the University of Liverpool, UK.

Kirsten Bell is a Research Associate in the Department of Anthropology at the University of British Columbia, Canada.

Carol Kingdon is a Senior Research Fellow in the School of Health at the University of Central Lancashire, UK.

SOCIAL AND CULTURAL PERSPECTIVES ON HEALTH, TECHNOLOGY AND MEDICINE: OLD CONCEPTS, NEW PROBLEMS

Ciara Kierans, Kirsten Bell and Carol Kingdon

Routledge
Taylor & Francis Group
LONDON AND NEW YORK

First edition published 2016
by Routledge
2 Park Square, Milton Park, Abingdon, Oxon OX14 4RN

Simultaneously published in the USA and Canada
by Routledge
711 Third Avenue, New York, NY 10017

Routledge is an imprint of the Taylor & Francis Group, an informa business

British Library Cataloguing in Publication Data
A catalogue record for this book is available from the British Library

Library of Congress Cataloguing in Publication Data
A catalog record for this book has been requested

ISBN: 978-1-138-94108-3 (hbk)
ISBN: 978-1-138-94110-6 (pbk)
ISBN: 978-1-315-67388-2 (ebk)

Typeset in Bembo
by Out of House Publishing

MIX
Paper from responsible sources
FSC www.fsc.org FSC® C013056

Printed and bound in Great Britain by
TJ International Ltd, Padstow, Cornwall

CONTENTS

FIGURES AND TABLES

Figures

Tables

FOREWORD

As someone who majored as an undergraduate in both sociology and anthropology, I have often felt that these two disciplines are rather arbitrarily and unnecessarily separate from each other. I then went on to complete a professional public health higher degree (a Master's of Public Health) followed by a doctorate within public health in a Faculty of Medicine that brought sociology and media and cultural studies to bear on a medical condition (HIV/AIDS). It became more apparent to me that interdisciplinary sociocultural perspectives on health and medical issues were vitally important. When studying such topics as epidemiology, health promotion and health economics during the Master's degree, my training in sociology and anthropology provoked me to challenge and question the taken-for-granted norms and assumptions that underpinned them.

Since then, I have made it one of my academic missions to view biomedicine and public health through a sociocultural lens, identifying the assemblages of humans, knowledges, beliefs, discourses, practices and technologies that underpin them. Although I identify predominantly as a sociologist, I have benefited hugely from including anthropological research and theory in my own research, as well as incorporating the perspectives offered by media and cultural studies, science and technology studies and cultural geography. One of my first books, *Medicine as Culture*, was given this title to highlight the notion of biomedicine as a cultural artefact. In developing the arguments in the book I drew on the work of several medical anthropologists. The redoubtable British cultural anthropologist Mary Douglas has remained one of my favourite scholars, and I have used her work to theorise topics as diverse as risk, eating habits, obesity politics, infant embodiment and self-tracking practices.

To fail to acknowledge the interesting insights offered by other disciplines or sub-disciplines is short-sighted and ultimately impoverishes one's research and theorizing. Yet books that bring together sociology and anthropology to highlight the social and cultural dimensions of biomedicine remain rare. This book represents one such attempt, with Ciara Kierans and Kirsten Bell, as medical anthropologists, collaborating with sociologist Carol Kingdon. The book brings what the authors describe as 'old concepts' to bear in explaining elements of the use of technologies in biomedicine that are not always immediately apparent. Kierans, Bell and Kingdon use traditionally anthropological concepts such as culture, ritual, kinship, magic, the gift and exchange to identify these elements. Some of these concepts are rarely employed in sociological accounts of biomedicine and technology. This book represents an important step forward in demonstrating their use and value.

Renowned anthropological scholars are often excluded in medical sociology, as are sociological thinkers from medical anthropology. Furthermore, medical sociology, in its focus on the developed world, often fails to incorporate cross-cultural perspectives that can do much to highlight the cultural relativity of ideas of medicine, health and illness. This book is able to demonstrate the ways in which each discipline has something to offer the other. The overviews that are provided in each chapter of the histories of research related to the concepts and scholars on which they centre are excellent introductions. Each chapter then goes on to demonstrate the relevance of this scholarship to understanding biomedicine and technology.

The authors also combine their anthropological and sociological sensibilities to write a final chapter on the body, a topic that has received a high level of interest in both sociology and anthropology, particularly in the 1990s and early 2000s (the key journal on this topic, *Body & Society*, was launched in 1995). The sociology and anthropology of the body appear to have lost some popularity over the past decade. It is difficult to understand why this is the case, save for recognizing the effect of academic vogues – topics and theorists come into fashion and then go out again as new topics and theorists take their place. Yet the body, in conjunction with selfhood, identity and social relations, remains a central topic of importance for the social sciences, and of vital interest to sociocultural studies of medicine. This point is emphasized not only in the concluding chapter of the book but all the way through; after all, all forms of medicine are always about human bodies.

What next for the sociology and anthropology of biomedicine and technology? I would hazard a guess that critical data studies will become an increasingly important area of research for both disciplines, as medicine becomes colonized by digital health technologies and both healthcare professionals and the lay public are faced with making sense of the continuous flows of digital data that many of these devices generate. Many of the discussions in this book are highly relevant to a critical analysis of digital health. For example, nowhere is magical thinking more apparent than in the techno-utopian visions of the potentially 'disruptive' potential of social media and self-tracking digital devices and the investment of faith and trust in the apparently 'neutral' and large-scale knowledges offered by big data in medicine and public health. The new 'sexy profession' of data science offers rituals for this particular magic. Instead of talking about the 'cyborg body', we might now refer to the 'digitized data assemblage' that is configured from the entanglements of digital technologies, digital data and human flesh. More than ever we will need anthropological and sociological scholarship to make provocations and interventions into this world of novel technologies in biomedicine.

Deborah Lupton, Centenary Research Professor, News & Media Research Centre, Faculty of Arts & Design, University of Canberra

ACKNOWLEDGEMENTS

We would like to thank Deborah Lupton for taking time out of her busy schedule to write the Foreword. We are also very grateful to our editor, Katherine Ong, for her support of the manuscript. The three anonymous reviewers of our book proposal also provided helpful feedback that enabled us to refine the scope of the book and exactly what it was we were trying to accomplish with it. The book itself has had a complicated and lengthy gestation over a number of years. We would therefore like to acknowledge Elizabeth Ettorre and Jude Robinson, both of whom were involved in this project at various points, although not part of the book's final iteration.

Ciara would like to thank her partner, colleague and collaborator, Michael Mair, for his steadfast academic and personal support on this project as a whole and, in particular, his scholarly advice and careful editorial eye on the culture, exchange and body chapters. Sincere thanks also to fellow anthropologists Mark Maguire and Jane Parish for their careful readings of and counsel on the exchange chapter, to colleagues Susan Pickard and Bethan Evans for their feedback and suggestions on the body chapter and similarly to Helen Keane for providing valuable insight also on the body chapter.

Kirsten is indebted to Bruce Kapferer, who had a formative influence on her thinking as an anthropologist and who kindly agreed to give feedback on the magic chapter, along with her colleagues Simone Dennis and Vinay Kamat. She is also very grateful to Bill McKellin and Kieran O'Doherty for their comments on the kinship chapter, which saved her from several embarrassing gaffs (any remaining ones she takes full responsibility for). Likewise, Helen Keane was kind enough to provide speedy feedback on the body chapter and her expert eye was greatly appreciated. Finally, she thanks Andrew Ham, who got to observe the highs and lows of this project from close quarters and provided sage counsel throughout.

Carol would like to thank Michael Mair and Gayle Letherby, who provided expert reviews on chapter drafts. She would also like to thank Soo Downe at the University of Central Lancashire, Zarko Alfirevic and Kim Hall at the University of Liverpool, and clinical colleagues at Liverpool Women's Hospital. Gracious thanks also must go to Sheila Crowder, Linda Barr and Lorna Edwards, who made her contributions possible in more ways than they know; her husband, Martin Flanagan; and her daughter, Niamh – who is world-making in so many ways.

INTRODUCTION

For some time now, developments in science, health, and technology have provided fertile analytical ground for social science disciplines such as anthropology and sociology. Recent thinking in these fields has helped to illustrate how shifts in medical and scientific knowledge continue to give new life to old debates about the relations between society, culture, knowledge and the individual. These debates raise questions about the particular role of the social sciences in tracking and making sense of these developments.

By way of example, in a 2013 polemic published in the *New York Times*, Nicholas Christakis, a medical practitioner and sociologist, argued that the social sciences need a shake-up. He contends that they have become conservative, lacking in innovation, weak in multidisciplinarity and are failing to address the big issues of our times, unlike our colleagues in the natural sciences – particularly those in the fields of systems biology, neurobiology and molecular physics. Commenting on Christakis' arguments, Amanda Goodall and Andrew Oswald, both social scientists, broadly concurred with his assessment, suggesting that what 'principally matters is whether social scientists are doing their job of helping humans to understand the world and improve it' (Goodall and Oswald, 2014). The range of controversies that such critiques set in motion are far from new; they are a response to the pressures placed on the social sciences today to produce more 'impact', to be more translatable and more transformative. For our present purposes, they also reveal the resurfacing of longstanding assumptions about the proper role and applications of social science research and thinking as it engages with topics in medicine, science and technology.

At the core of Christakis, Goodall and Oswald's position is the assumption that the job of the social sciences is to study 'problems' as they are established or formulated by the natural sciences. In the context of such formulations, this means that the work social scientists do is consigned to the 'downstream' consequences of scientific developments – a doctrine that limits social science to the study of what has come to be known as 'ELSI': the ethical, legal and social implications of science.[1] Many, however, have resisted this assessment, challenging the idea that the social scientist is best seen as an under-labourer working on behalf of the natural sciences, assisting them to more effectively see their projects through.

Those unwilling to take on the mantle of under-labourer question the separation of the technical or 'natural' and the social as different orders of knowledge and practice. This has led to a growing body of work subjecting the 'upstream' technical production of scientific knowledge *in* scientific practice to sustained, empirically grounded critical appraisal. Such research illustrates that the concerns of science, per se, are not simply outcomes of nature and technology but also products of institutional, cultural, political and epistemological arrangements. In contrast to the stories told by medicine, science and technology about their own operations, social scientists have shown that where we do subject scientific practice to empirical study, we see a non-linear process of development. Discontinuities and breaks are the norm, instead of continuity and simple progression. Ideas re-emerge and are reshuffled and recycled in different places and times; they are reworked in different registers, rhetorics and with different politics.

Innovations in genetic therapies, advanced pharmaceutical interventions, surgical techniques and personalized medicine, to name but a few, have resurrected a (re) turn to positivism, behaviourism, sociobiology, liberal debates on the 'ownership of the self', as well as ahistorical/acontextual recalibrations of population, racial and socioeconomic differences. In other words, transformations in science and technology have reanimated much older controversies, sites of interpretive conflict and disputes over how best to think about the relationship between society and nature – including ways of thinking we may have thought were consigned to history. As a result of these developments, it is crucial to examine our analytical, methodological and theoretical resources – those that help to weigh up, understand and make sense of the interlinkages between science and society.

Our agenda

Social and Cultural Perspectives on Health, Technology and Medicine: Old Concepts, New Problems represents one attempt at such an examination. Our starting premise is that the different forms of social and cultural inquiry that have developed since the mid-nineteenth century in the fields of anthropology and sociology provide us with a key stock of conceptual resources for understanding and interrogating developments in medicine, science and technology. We are particularly interested in the manner in which some of our most enduring core concepts – culture, society, magic, production, kinship, exchange and the body – have been taken up, made to work and have come to be reworked across the natural and social sciences. Indeed, the fact that they *have* been so widely taken up is evidence of precisely the 'impact' of the social sciences that is so intensely decried in the current moment, although it is admittedly of a rather different order to that of the natural sciences.

Steven Shapin (1995) observes that unlike the knowledge natural scientists produce, the credibility of concepts and phenomena in the human and social sciences depends less on their authorization by specialists and more on the extent to which they are vernacularized:

> the extent to which they actually come to constitute the phenomenal base to which they refer. If people, as it appears many of them now do, make sense of their lives by organizing them with respect to such notions, to that extent... human science has regenerated and recreated *human nature*.
>
> (Shapin, 1995: 267, emphasis in original)

The fact that 'cultural competence' training is now commonplace within medical education (Taylor, 2003), public health clinicians readily speak of 'the social determinants of health' (Raphael, 2011) and oncologists comment on 'magical thinking' among patients (Salander, 2000) is evidence of just how widely these concepts have travelled. As such examples illustrate, social scientists have disseminated our core concepts 'as effectively as utility companies deliver electricity and telephone services' (Latour, 2005: 4).

In documenting their journeys, we ask the following questions: What are their enduring features? What are their methodological and analytical possibilities and constraints? How are they contested and by whom? How have they been employed (and deployed) inside and outside of our disciplines? In exploring these questions, we aim to demonstrate the contemporary value of these conceptual heritages, drawing together both old and new ways of thinking. Our goal is also to situate the disciplines of anthropology and sociology as critical interlocutors *within* rather than *at the margins of* contemporary scientific developments. In recognition of the different ways in which the work of the social sciences 'extends' over time and space through dialogue and convergence between disciplines (Osborne and Rose, 1999), we show that older concepts, when appropriately contextualized, retain considerable relevance for social scientists and health scholars seeking to make sense of medicine, science and technology and the problems that surround them today.

In working with these concepts, our goal is most decidedly *not* to provide a Whiggish or canonical account that traces their unilineal 'development' and the march of epistemic progress through time, with the past judged through the lens of the present. Indeed, if this book shows one thing, it is that the concepts we draw on have always been complex and contested – earlier scholars were often far more aware of the limitations of their uses than we give them credit for today. While the postmodern, postcolonial turn has sometimes led to a tendency to dismiss earlier scholarship, one of the underlying motivations for this book is our belief that there is much that is of value in these early theories and debates, that the past and the present continue to interact (Benjamin, 1999), and that the issues and concerns that preoccupied these scholars are still very much alive today. While it is easy to look back upon this work and see everything that is wrong with it – from the sexism and racism of its language, to the sometimes problematic assumptions underpinning it – as Maurice Merleau-Ponty (1964: 109) observed, 'we are all hemmed in by history'. Thus, 'whatever truth we may have is to be gotten not in spite of but through our historical inherence'.

Our orientation is, therefore, to keep in view the interactions of past and present. In so doing, we aim to explicate the intersections between the concepts we explore and their cross-fertilizations. Perhaps a little unusually for a co-authored book, the chapters are individually authored, bar the final one on the body. We have taken this approach because the chapters play to our individual research strengths and interests. Although we have made use of our own empirical work to varying degrees, the case studies have all been informed by our respective research programmes. Each chapter includes an overview of the core concept, its salience to the fields of health, technology and medicine, and empirical examples and case studies through which we organize and ground our examination. The illustrative case studies reflect our shared emphasis on medical technologies in our work (e.g., genetic technologies, reproductive technologies, transplant technologies, imaging technologies) and medical problems (organ failure, cancer, stillbirth, addiction) as especially productive sites for exploring key concepts and the debates they have generated.

Although we believe that the concepts we have chosen to explore provide foundational 'equipment for thinking',[2] any attempt to single out core concepts will always be susceptible to the charge of omission. We are therefore acutely aware that there are numerous others that we might have explored: race, ethnicity, gender, the self, the state, power, for example; although issues relating to these concepts do emerge in many of the chapters. We have also been necessarily selective in the scholarship we have chosen to focus on in each chapter and our examinations should not be taken as comprehensive summaries (there are plenty of books and articles that present these). Our goal is perhaps best described as one that privileges the *use* of concepts rather than asserting what they do or should mean. We signpost for the reader the broader landscape of research within which they can navigate for their own means and ends.

Core concepts and disciplinary boundaries

By focusing on concepts, our goal was to transcend disciplinary boundaries to map the ways they have been taken up *across* disciplines and fields. However, it is indisputably the case that most have been claimed more by one discipline than the other – and this is evident in the relative weighting placed upon anthropological versus sociological scholarship in a number of chapters.[3] Although the proclaimed disciplinary boundaries between anthropology and sociology may be largely rhetorical in character (Fuller, 1991), they are nevertheless meaningful in terms of how each discipline came to construct itself and its central project. Thus, if sociology and anthropology are 'imagined communities' (Anderson, 1983), like other such communities they have their own mythologies, stocks of knowledge and ancestral heroes. In situating our concepts, we draw out the contributions of such 'ancestral heroes' and the role they have played in generating conceptual tools *and* the disciplinary frameworks they acquired relevance within. Although several figures have exerted enormous influence on both disciplines (e.g., Karl Marx, Max Weber and Émile Durkheim), and there are certain scholars they lay equal claim to (most notably Pierre Bourdieu), others we regard as specific to each. For example, E.E. Evans-Pritchard and Bronisław Malinowski might be staples of undergraduate anthropology courses, but rare is the sociology curriculum that covers them; likewise, key sociologists such as C. Wright Mills and Norbert Elias seldom surface for the undergraduate student in anthropology.

Our disciplinary canons also differ in the types of issues and questions they have historically addressed. Although sometimes the differences between the two disciplines have been glossed in terms of a 'West versus the rest' or 'us versus the other' divide, as Rena Lederman (2004) notes, anthropologists have always studied people everywhere.[4] This is also true of sociologists, as the work of key figures such as Émile Durkheim and Marcel Mauss attests. Instead, it might be more accurate to say that sociocultural anthropology historically had a focus on the exotic (Kapferer, 2012).[5] Sociology, on the other hand, while equally interested in challenging dominant modes of thought and 'common-sense' assumptions about the world, had a different mode of entry into such topics, focusing instead on social institutions and social structures.

A third difference between the two disciplines is a methodological one, with anthropology much more strongly associated with what Kapferer (2007: 81) terms the 'ethnographic imperative'. Indeed, this is perhaps their critical difference. As Steve Fuller (1991: 302) observes: 'Disciplines mark the point at which methods are institutionalized, or so to speak, the world is made flesh'. According to Kapferer (2007), a central feature of anthropology as an Enlightenment project was the stress placed on the ethnographic over the conceptual, interpretational and abstract. While numerous sociologists conduct ethnographic research, in the discipline it tends to be treated more as a discrete research method as opposed to an underlying *raison d'être* (see Lederman, 2004).

However, it was not until the twentieth-century period of professionalization (especially following World War I) that ethnographic fieldwork became the hallmark of anthropology. In the nineteenth and early twentieth century, the boundaries between the two disciplines (and others besides) were far more porous. Thus, it is fairly common for scholars writing in the earlier period to be claimed as both anthropologists and sociologists, and ethnologists and philosophers to boot – Herbert Spencer and Lucien Lévy-Bruhl are two cases in point. Even after disciplinary boundaries solidified, there continued to be a considerable degree of crossover between anthropological and sociological writings and the intellectual paradigms that influenced both disciplines. Indeed, all disciplines are 'constantly influenced by points of view and methods of related disciplines' (Thompson Klein, 1993: 186), even as they define themselves against them.

Work across the social sciences, past and present, shows that methodological traditions regularly overlap and converge and the supposedly discrete dividing lines between disciplines have always been subject to blurring that gives rise to heterogeneous and multi-sited practices. The interdisciplinary domain of science and technology studies is one arena in which these shared intellectual heritages, among others, can clearly be seen. As a hybrid field consisting of anthropologists, sociologists, philosophers, legal scholars and historians united by an interest in the cultural, historical and social contexts of science and technology, various key figures in science and technology studies elude disciplinary capture and many traverse disciplinary boundaries with ease. For example, Bruno Latour is frequently characterized as a philosopher, anthropologist and sociologist.

Such intertwining can also been seen in the range of debates that shaped and reshaped thinking in the social sciences throughout the twentieth century. Debates on rationality, structural functionalism and so on occurred amid a series of interdisciplinary 'turns': rhetorical, literary, interpretive, Marxist, feminist, linguistic and practice-oriented. The influence of Marxist and feminist approaches, in particular, hold significance for many of the chapters in this book (see Chapters 2, 4, 5, 6 and 7). As Julie Thompson Klein (1993) notes, these larger shifts impacted the social sciences from the 1970s onwards, each signalling the widespread dissatisfaction with positivist models of knowledge and naïve theories of representation, serving to further blur the boundaries between disciplines. In her words: 'In the wake of these debates "blurred genres" became a metaphor of the times, a ready signifier of the growing number of cross-disciplinary borrowings, projects, and new categories of knowledge that document increased permeation of disciplinary boundaries' (Thompson Klein, 1993: 187). Thus, as with other imagined communities, while most of us identify strongly with one discipline or the other, the differences between them are clearly less great – certainly less absolute – than we often assert.

Although disciplinary boundaries continue to be marked and policed in various ways, it is also worth bearing in mind that in health and medical contexts, the 'social scientist' versus 'non-social scientist' divide is arguably more salient than disciplinary distinctions themselves. Many health professionals and researchers trained outside of the social sciences perceive little difference between the two disciplines. Moreover, anthropologists and sociologists working in departments of health and medicine may find that disciplinary distinctions fade largely to irrelevance in the face of their minority status. At the same time, as more health professionals take postgraduate courses with very specific anthropological and sociological content, or collaborate with social scientists on a day-to-day basis, disciplinary distinctions become salient once more in the kinds of research questions posed and incorporated into new transdisciplinary projects.

For this and other reasons, in this book we are not trying to defend disciplinary or territorial boundaries. Nevertheless, returning to core concepts enables us to productively see anthropology and sociology as laboratories for innovation, explication and critique that have generated resources for thinking about the social, cultural and political aspects of the worlds that we inhabit. Furthermore, in focusing on a subject matter that is in large part forged in, through and by science, medicine and technology, we aim to share with readers those particular approaches we have found most useful in opening up these domains as sites for research and the conceptual approaches that have enabled us to do so.

Overview of chapters

Culture, the focus of Chapter 1, although widely drawn on across many fields of knowledge, is arguably anthropology's principal and most enduring interpretive 'tool' *and* its most contested. The culture concept has been extensively critiqued within and outside of the discipline, with little resolution or consensus over its meaning, utility and durability. In tracing culture's legacy since the late nineteenth century to the present day, Ciara draws out a series of theoretical and methodological debates that show culture to be not simply a device used to explicate the similarities and differences of various peoples and their practices, but also a *field* of practice. It is an arena where different thinkers and groups of thinkers manoeuvre, interact and come to occupy positions relative to one another through the ways in which they mobilize culture to do certain things.

Demonstrating the changing landscape of anthropological scholarship, this chapter achieves three things. First, it provides an overview of the concept's meandering career in anthropology. Second, it examines the ways in which it has been invoked, taken up and put to use outside of anthropology, demonstrating its problematic status as an explanatory variable for health and medicine. Finally, and with reference to ethnographic cases on transplant medicine and its cultural encounters, the chapter offers alternative ways of working with the concept, by positioning culture as an outcome or endpoint of social processes.

Chapter 2 traces the various trajectories taken by the **society** concept. It asserts that what is most interesting about society is *how* people live together and with what consequences. This outwardly simple idea is shown to have tasked sociologists from the formation of sociology as a discipline to the present day. Among others, the chapter draws from the writings of Émile Durkheim at the end of the nineteenth century, whose work offers an anchor point for the chapter as a whole. Questions of why society is important, how it is held together, made and remade, and what the relationship is between the individual and society, are highlighted as enduring concerns for social science scholars grappling with the complexity of modernity and social change. Carol shows that while some sociologists have turned away from society as a conceptual resource, it has gained prominence elsewhere, such as in the particular (positivist) vision of the social advanced through 'social determinants' discourses in public health medicine.

The chapter argues for a return to the concept of society in all its guises to advance cross-disciplinary agendas for health. Stillbirth is used as a case study to tease out the present-day utility of society as a conceptual resource that is broader than how it is conceptualized through and by the social determinants of health framework. In doing so, the chapter aims to achieve three things. First, it demonstrates how society has been taken up by social scientists, the relationships between these positions, and their promise. Second, it shows how a particular vision of the social has been employed in the field of public health, which is both partial and problematic. Third and finally, it highlights the promise of the concept when taken as multiple.

Chapter 3 explores the preoccupation with questions of causality that has driven anthropological research into **magic**. This topic is particularly salient for studies of health and medicine because of the split biomedicine presumes between science and magic, with the former category rational and instrumental and the latter irrational and symbolic. Following a discussion of early theories on the relationship between magic, religion and science espoused by Sir James Frazer, Émile Durkheim and Lucien Lévy-Bruhl, Kirsten focuses on three particularly influential figures in the study of magic – Bronisław Malinowski, E.E. Evans-Pritchard and Claude Lévi-Strauss – and the ways in which the ethnographic realities they engaged with exceeded their theories. To varying degrees, such work challenged the distinctions between the natural and supernatural, the symbolic and instrumental, and science and magic.

Unfortunately, these dualisms continued to plague studies of ritual, which emerged as primary conceptual terrain from the 1950s. However, the work ofVictor Turner was integral in illuminating the ways in which ritual is both instrumental and symbolic – how ritual might *do* things in the 'real' world. Kirsten argues that this insight is critical to understanding the placebo effect, a phenomenon that challenges biomedicine's conceptualization of cause and effect. Through a case study on lay understandings of causality about cancer and cancer treatment, she advocates the need to move beyond the dualisms that continue to pervade understandings of health and illness and biomedicine and 'ethnomedicine'.

Chapter 4 focuses on the **production** concept as a means to understanding the character of social relations in different societies. In the first part of the chapter, Carol traces the co-constituted conceptual heritages of production and consumption from Karl Marx to the present day, including how they have been taken up in theories on 'medicalization' and 'biomedicalization'. Through these literatures, the concepts are shown to be especially relevant to the shifting boundaries between the hitherto curative practices of medicine, and the present-day trend for enhancement of life, lifestyle and self-identity through medicine.

The chapter then demonstrates how feminist scholarship has reconceived production in relation to reproduction and reproductive technologies. In recent decades, the reproductive body (male and female) has become increasingly commercialized and rendered perfectible through science, medicine, technology, the market and the media, with demand, health and healthcare consequences purportedly a matter of individual choice. Through a case study of childbirth, and planned caesarean birth in particular, Carol shows how capitalism penetrates and transforms so-called 'natural' processes, technologies and healthcare.

Once virtually synonymous with the discipline of anthropology, the concept of **kinship** is the focus of Chapter 5. Anthropologists were always aware that kinship was something more than an expression of blood relationships. However, what kinship was and how it should be approached was the source of ongoing debate in the discipline, and one key means through which the battle lines between various intellectual paradigms (e.g., structural functionalism and structuralism) were drawn. Taking the reader through the critiques of kinship that markedly intensified from the 1970s, Kirsten shows their connection with broader shifts in anthropology – especially the growing influence of feminist anthropology and the postcolonial critiques of the discipline.

She illustrates that the primary outcome of such scholarship was a denaturalization of kinship, wherein it was unmoored from its prior grounding in notions of blood and biogenesis. However, integral to this process of denaturalization was the rise of reproductive and genetic technologies, both of which have blurred the boundaries between what can be attributed to nature and culture. Through a case study on genetic cancer counselling, Kirsten explores the ways in which kinship is currently being enacted in this setting. As she illustrates, kinship is a primary site wherein notions of what counts as natural and cultural continue to be articulated.

Chapter 6 is concerned with developments in technology and medicine and the ways in which the mechanisms of **exchange** underpin their growth and expansion. Organized around the trope of *The Gift* – the seminal work of Marcel Mauss – and its juxtaposition with commodity frameworks, Ciara traces their significance and critical limitations as analytical determinants for modes of bodily transfer. Drawing on empirical work on tissue, blood and whole body exchange, she emphasizes the importance of focusing our efforts on the ways in which the body and its parts function as sites for enacting of various modes of exchange, rather than the other way around. This opens up a more nuanced set of understandings that enables us to detail the interrelationship between issues of obligation, interest, entitlement, status, altruism, the desire to contribute to knowledge – scientific and social – and therapeutic wellbeing.

Modes of exchange, such as gift-giving, reciprocal transfers and buying and selling, are complex social arrangements that establish and sustain social relations. Deeply reflective of the social and cultural fabric out of which they are formed, modes of exchange are simultaneously pragmatic and symbolic exercises. They are central to our understandings of the variable interrelationship between things, people and power and so provide significant interpretive value for the disciplines of anthropology and sociology.

Finally, in Chapter 7, Ciara and Kirsten focus on the **body**. The body has emerged within the social sciences as a vital analytical resource, one that opens up and mobilizes debates across medicine, science and society. Recent scholarship has shown the body to operate less as a concept in itself, and more as a site for the production of concepts – concepts that are fundamental to theorizing the arrangements and social relations of contemporary life. A critical site for rethinking power and difference, a symbolic analogue of social formation, an existential ground for the production of culture and the self, thinking on and with the body serves to link domains that are often kept apart and so provides a uniting heuristic for the previous six chapters. Working with an idea of the 'embodied subject', we map out three key interlinking modalities of bodily thought and practice: the body as 'lived'; 'disciplined' and 'classified'. Although far from exhaustive, these orientations open up different ways of thinking about the status of the body – living and dead – theoretically and methodologically, across time and disciplinary endeavour. In this way, we show the analytical significance of the body-as-concept to be essential to our rethinking the relationship between medicine, technology and society. We conclude with reference to an exemplar case study on addiction and the growth of neuroscientific approaches that treat addiction as a disease of the brain. This example helps to tease out the complex over-layering of methodological positions on the body as object, construct and sentient subject.

Notes

1 For critiques of ELSI see Rabinow and Bennett (2012) on designing human practices.
2 We are paraphrasing Burke (1957) and Blum (2015).
3 Undoubtedly, our own disciplinary backgrounds (Ciara and Kirsten were trained in social anthropology and Carol in sociology) have also informed our readings.
4 This view also arises out of an assumed isomorphism of space, place and culture that Gupta and Ferguson (1992) have strongly critiqued.
5 As Kapferer (2012) observes, while this orientation has come under sustained attack both from within and outside the discipline, there is a certain sense in which a reconfigured notion of the exotic (stripped of its emphasis on essence and associated dualisms) continues to be central to anthropology. After all, 'everything and anything is potentially in an exotic relation. Nothing is intrinsically exotic except through the relations into which it is drawn' (Kapferer, 2012: 815).

References

Anderson, B. (1983) *Imagined Communities: Reflections on the Origin and Spread of Nationalism*. London: Verso.

Benjamin, W. (1999) *The Arcades Project*. Translated by H. Eiland and K. McLaughlin. Cambridge, MA: Belknap Press.

Blum, A. (2015) Guide(s) for the perplexed: science and literature as equipment for living. *Philosophy and Rhetoric*, 48(1): 54–72.

Burke, K. (1957) *The Philosophy of Literary Form*. Berkeley, CA: University of California Press.

Christakis, N.A. (2013) Let's shake up the social sciences. *New York Times*. Available at: www.nytimes.com/2013/07/21/opinion/sunday/lets-shake-up-the-social-sciences.html.

Fuller, S. (1991) Disciplinary boundaries and the rhetoric of the social sciences. *Poetics Today*, 12(2): 301–325.

Goodall, A. and Oswald, A. (2014) Do the social sciences need a shake up? *Times Higher Education*. Available at: www.timeshighereducation.co.uk/features/do-the-social-sciences-need-a-shake-up/2016165.fullarticle.

Gupta, A. and Ferguson, J. (1992) Beyond 'culture': space, identity, and the politics of difference. *Cultural Anthropology*, 7(1): 6–23.

Kapferer, B. (2007) Anthropology and the dialectic of the Enlightenment: a discourse on the definition and ideals of a threatened discipline. *The Australian Journal of Anthropology*, 18(1): 72–96.

Kapferer, B. (2012) How anthropologists think: configurations of the exotic. *Journal of the Royal Anthropological Institute*, 19: 813–836.

Latour, B. (2005) *Reassembling the Social: An Introduction to Actor-Network-Theory*. Oxford: Oxford University Press.

Lederman, R. (2004) Towards an anthropology of disciplinarity. *Critical Matrix*, 15: 60–68.

Merleau-Ponty, M. (1964) *Signs*. Evanston, IL: Northwestern University Press.

Osborne, T. and Rose, N. (1999) Do the social sciences create phenomena? The example of public opinion research. *The British Journal of Sociology*, 50: 367–396.

Rabinow, P. and Bennett, G. (2012) *Designing Human Practices: an Experiment with Synthetic Biology*. Chicago, IL: University of Chicago Press.

Raphael, D. (2011) A discourse analysis of the social determinants of health. *Critical Public Health*, 21(2): 221–236

Salander, P. (2000) Using beliefs and magical thinking to fight cancer distress: a case study. *Psycho-Oncology*, 9(1): 40–43.

Shapin, S. (1995) Cordelia's love: credibility and the social studies of science. *Perspectives on Science*, 3(3): 255–275.

Taylor, J. (2003) Confronting 'culture' in medicine's 'culture of no culture'. *Academic Medicine*, 78(6): 555–559.

Thompson Klein, J. (1993) Blurring, cracking, and crossing: permeation and the fracturing of discipline. In E. Messer-Davidow, D.R. Shumway and D.J. Sylvan (eds.), *Knowledges: Historical and Critical Studies in Disciplinarity*. Charlottesville, VA: University of Virginia Press, 185–213.

1

CULTURE

Ciara Kierans

> Culture is a deeply compromised idea I cannot yet do without.
>
> James Clifford, *The Predicament of Culture*

Introduction

If we can agree on one thing within the discipline of anthropology today with regard to the vexed concept of culture, it is what culture is not. Culture is *not* the sort of concept that can be pressed into a prescriptive role, reduced to sets of traits or understood as a causative agent. Phenomena associated with culture, such as beliefs, practices, symbols and so on, are not free-floating, abstracted features of everyday life. Nor is culture simply the property of a group. What it *does* constitute, however, is a different story. Anthropologists, who use culture as their principal interpretive tool, readily admit its contested and changing character. It has been extensively critiqued within the discipline, most intensively over the past 30 years, with little resolution or consensus over its long-term durability or utility (Frankenberg, 1995). It is possibly best characterized by the shifting discourses that have underpinned various attempts to define it, definitions that pinball between its objectivist, symbolic, discursive and practised referents.

Michael Agar, borrowing from Roy D'Andrade, gets straight to the heart of the matter:

> Culture is a mess, akin to 'studying snow in the middle of an avalanche'. You can see why some argue that we should consider dropping the word from our vocabulary. This will never happen, though, since anthropology only gets one vote in the crowded marketplace of global discourse, and global discourse is enamoured of the term culture and isn't about to give it up. For now let's

> continue with culture, continue to redefine the concept so that we can say 'culture means this', even if we know what we say has the chance of the proverbial snowball in hell of ever influencing popular uses of the term.
>
> (Agar, 2006: 5)

In the spirit of such refined resignation, this chapter attempts to do three things: (1) to provide an overview of the concept's meandering career in anthropology; (2) to examine its position in the 'crowded marketplace of global discourse' by empirically demonstrating culture as a 'topic of concern' for health and medicine; and (3) to consider ways in which we might continue to work with the concept. Although far from offering any prescription for its use, I hope what follows will stand as a resource for students and researchers who are interested in the concept, one that might aid navigation of the anthropological terrain.

Reflections upon culture at the crash-points of disciplinary inquiry

There are, in anthropology, an abundance of reviews that have sought to map out trajectories of the culture concept over much of the twentieth century (see Elias, 1978 [1939]; Kroeber and Kluckhohn, 1952; Stocking, 1966; Harris, 1968; Ortner, 1984; Clifford and Marcus, 1986; Kuper, 1999). While there are benefits to tracing the progression of a concept, it's equally important not to assume historical developments represent intellectual advancements. Adam Kuper's treatment of the work of culture in anthropology cautions:

> Modern arguments [over culture] do not precisely recapitulate earlier controversies... Each generation modernises the idiom of debate, usually adapting it to current scientific terminology; evolutionism in the late 19th century, organicism in the early 20th century, relativity in the 1920s.
>
> (Kuper, 1999: 9)

As a consequence, explications of culture and the various definitional disputes that have accompanied them might best be thought of as a *field* of practice in Pierre Bourdieu's sense of the term: an arena where different thinkers and groups of thinkers manoeuvre, interact and come to occupy positions relative to one another through the ways in which they mobilize culture to do certain things. Culture is a term that has been employed to denote national identities as much as disciplinary objects and boundaries. It has been at the very heart of anthropology as a discipline. If culture has been drawn on to understand distinctions, we also must recognize that it has emerged as a product *of* distinctions (Bourdieu, 1984). That is, the ways in which anthropologists have taken up the concept are themselves connected to wider uses and ways of marking difference. The following section presents an overview of key points in the concept's career. They are drawn on only to anchor the changing and contested terrain of culture and are in no way comprehensive. Definitions of culture advanced by some of the authors cited in this next section can be found in Table 1.

TABLE 1 Definitions of culture

1.1 Edward Burnett Tylor (1958 [1871]: 1)	Culture, or civilization, taken in its broad, ethnographic sense, is that complex whole which includes knowledge, belief, art, morals, law, custom, and any other capabilities and habits acquired by man as a member of society.
1.2 Franz Boas (1911: 149)	Culture may be defined as the totality of the mental and physical reactions and activities that characterize the behavior of individuals composing a social group collectively and individually in relation to their natural environment, to other groups, to members of the group itself and of each individual to himself. It also includes the products of these activities and their role in the life of the groups. The mere enumerations of these various aspects of life, however, does not constitute culture. It is more, for its elements are not independent, they have a structure.
1.3 Margaret Mead (1937: 17)	Culture means the whole complex of traditional behavior which has been developed by the human race and is successively learned by each generation. A culture is less precise. It can mean the forms of traditional behavior which are characteristics of a given society, or of a group of societies, or of a certain race, or of a certain area, or of a certain period of time.
1.4 Bronisław Malinowski (1931: 623)	Culture is a well-organized unity divided into two fundamental aspects – a body of artifacts and a system of customs.
1.5 Ruth Benedict (1934: 16)	What really binds men together is their culture, … the ideas and the standards they have in common.
1.6 A.R. Radcliffe-Brown (1940: 2)	We do not observe a 'culture', since that word denotes, not any concrete reality, but an abstraction, and as it is commonly used a vague abstraction. But direct observation does reveal to us that these human beings are connected by a complex network of social relations. I use the term 'social structure' to denote this network of actually existing relations.
1.7 Talcott Parsons (1951: 2)	Cultural objects are symbolic elements of the cultural tradition, ideas or beliefs, expressive symbols or value patterns.
1.8 Alfred Kroeber and Clyde Kluckhohn (1952: 357)	Culture consists of patterns, explicit and implicit, of and for behavior acquired and transmitted by symbols, constituting the distinctive achievements of human groups, including their embodiments in artifacts; the essential core of culture consists of traditional (i.e. historically derived and selected) ideas and especially their attached values; culture systems may, on the one hand, be considered as products of action, and on the other as conditioning elements of further action.
1.9 Clifford Geertz (1973: 5)	Man is an animal suspended in webs of significance he himself has spun. I take culture to be those webs, and the analysis of it to be therefore not an experimental science in search of law but an interpretative one in search of meaning.

1.10 Claude Lévi-Strauss (1969 [1949]: 4)	Man is a biological being as well as a social individual. Among the responses which he gives to external stimuli, some are the full product of his nature, and others of his condition... But it is not always easy to distinguish between the two... Culture is neither simply juxtaposed to nor simply superposed over life. In a way, culture substitutes itself to life, in another way culture uses and transforms life to realise a synthesis of a higher order.
1.11 James Clifford (1988: 19)	If culture is not an object to be described, neither is it a unified corpus of symbols and meanings that can be definitively interpreted. Culture is contested, temporal and emergent.
1.12 Paul Rabinow (1986: 241)	We do not need a theory of indigenous epistemologies or a new epistemology of the other. We should be attentive to our historical practice of projecting our cultural practices onto the other; at best, the task is to show how and when and through what cultural and institutional means other people started claiming epistemology for their own.

Culture: a modern construction

The contemporary anthropological use of culture emerged, post-Enlightenment, as an outcome of Europe's complex project of modernization. The Enlightenment had given rise to new social processes, institutions and discourses, engendering, in turn, new modes for thinking about oneself and one's place in a rapidly changing world (Porter, 2001). These new ways of thinking were, according to Norbert Elias, evident in the differences between what the French referred to as 'Civilization' and the Germans 'Kultur' (Elias, 1978 [1939]). 'Civilization', according to Elias, was explicitly an extension of the Enlightenment project. It manifested in pride in progress, in technological advancements, in the power of self-determining new societies and, in many respects, in the status of a newly modernized Europe as superior to other forms of society.

The German use of the term 'Zivilisation' similarly reflected these developments, but was ancillary to what they referred to as 'Kultur'. In this reading, Kultur, by comparison, is the expression or spirit of ordinary people, the outcome of history and tradition, visible in spiritual, artistic and creative endeavours. It is Kultur that establishes and delineates the ground of difference. For Elias (1978 [1939]: 8), 'it brought into focus those areas of the social life of humans which provided the politically excluded German middle classes with the main basis for their self-legitimization and the justification of their pride'. Kultur was, in fact, the bulwark against the immediate threats posed by Zivilisation: technological modernization and mass society (Gaughan and Lutzeier, 2007). Kultur, with its roots in the writing of the German philosopher Johann Gottfried Herder, is both political and social. In cohering a shared identity, it establishes a common and future path. The specific focus on the collective or 'lifeways' of a people, would have far-reaching consequences not only for German philosophers such as Friedrich Nietzsche and Wilhelm Dilthey, but also for Weber's methodological standpoint of 'verstehen'[1] and the rise of anthropology as a discipline (Kuper, 1999).

If conceptualizing culture became a way for the Germans to distinguish who they were in the changing economic and political landscape of nineteenth-century Europe, for many British thinkers it was a resource to enlarge understanding of an increasingly complex world, which included the expanding colonial territories and their place within them. That said, and echoing Grimshaw and Hart (1993: 21), we must be cautious not to 'indulge a parochial nationalism equating anthropology's development with specific histories', and so remain mindful that anthropological thought is diffuse and embedded in wider international projects. Nevertheless, colonial nations not only presented administrative problems to solve for an expanding British Empire, but generated new questions for intellectuals with regard to the visible diversity in social organization, social practice and physical form across the globe (Greenfield, 2001). Victorian thinkers such as Herbert Spencer and Sir James Frazer assumed that social differences could be constructed as a result of socially organized hierarchies, evolving as a logical consequence of natural competition. This crude evolutionary rendering laid the framework for the work of English anthropologist Edward Burnett Tylor's early fieldwork studies in Mexico and what would become anthropology's first formal definition of culture (Table 1.1).

Tylor's definition treated culture in unitary terms, with different societies progressing developmentally through time. Elaborated in *Primitive Culture* (1871), Tylor advocated that all cultures, past and present, must be studied as a part of a progressive history, moving from an animistic savage society to the modern civilized state. For many different reasons – political, commercial, intellectual and imperial – the idea of the Other was pushed into relief, and the concept of the 'primitive' took hold as a key organizational device in early anthropology (see Chapter 3), producing understandings of culture and naturalized orders of social division that, in turn, imposed classificatory arrangements that took the better part of the twentieth century to deconstruct.

It didn't take long before anthropologists were caught up in the contest to wrestle the concept from the scientific racism and discriminatory policies that inevitably followed on from evolutionary thinking. Initial efforts to disentangle culture from evolutionism are linked to the work of Franz Boas and his advancement of the theory of cultural relativism. Motivated by the writings of Rudolf Virchow (Stocking, 1974) and working among the Inuit, Boas questioned the classification and categorization of peoples according to evolutionary standards set by Western society. According to Boas, culture must be understood in the plural 'culture(s)' and within context (Stocking, 1966) (Table 1.2). Cultural relativism, therefore, advocated an understanding of culture on its own terms and in accordance with its own internal standards and values. For Boas, culture was learned, fundamentally a product of socialization and little rooted to biology. This approach was put to great effect by Boas's students, most influentially by Margaret Mead, whose 1928 monograph *Coming of Age in Samoa* stood as a testimony (albeit a problematic one[2]) to enduring nature/nurture or nature/culture debates (Table 1.3). Her work argued that the disturbances associated with adolescence in the US were not grounded in biological changes but were culturally shaped and ordered through childrearing and the values underpinning sexuality. Influentially, the Boasian tradition exercised the idea that evidence drawn from other cultures could be used to falsify generalized statements about the character of human behaviour, such as those proposed by biological determinists.

Building on the legacy of Boas, in addition to W.H.R. Rivers, Maurice Leenhardt and Marcel Mauss, to name only a few, Bronisław Malinowski furthered the relativist project and, in so doing, emphasized the importance of ethnographic fieldwork, as opposed to mere speculation, to capture what people do (Malinowski, 1922, 1927). Conducting fieldwork in north-western Melanesia, Malinowski proposed an understanding of cultural practice within the context of a social system's functioning, otherwise termed 'functionalism'. Culture, in other words, functions to meet the needs of individuals living with others, within a division of labour, which, in turn, enables their societies to operate in a systemic and coherent manner (Table 1.4). This bounded view of culture would later be subject to much critique in the discipline and beyond, owing to its homogenizing and ahistorical orientation. What Malinowski did achieve, however, was the carving out of a disciplinary niche, with sustained fieldwork cast as the hallmark of anthropology, a form of research integral to privileging the mundane and everyday over the extraordinary and exotic.

Looking back at Boas and Malinowski, it's clear that while a modernizing anthropology challenged the racialized hierarchies of the Victorians, it was dependent on small-scale society as the central unit of analysis. Theoretical expansion of the culture concept continued, as did the emergence of various schools of anthropology. In the US, Edward Sapir and his student Ruth Benedict broke with the Boasians, turning culture back towards original German conceptions (Table 1.5), and aligning it not only with broad national characteristics, but mapping those characteristics onto personality types and worldviews[3] (Benedict, 1934; Sapir, 1921). In the UK, A.R. Radcliffe-Brown, in a revision of Malinowski's functionalism and building upon Émile Durkheim's use of organicism (see Chapter 2), conceptualized culture in stronger interactional and structural terms, advocating a theory of structural functionalism (Table 1.6) as the route to understanding culture and its stabilization over time (Radcliffe-Brown, 1922). Taken together, the work of these early modern anthropologists laid the foundations for the expansion of social anthropology in UK universities, most notably the Manchester School through the work of Max Gluckman and his students; the anthropology department at the London School of Economics, by virtue of Bronisław Malinowski; and the department at Oxford University, which expanded under A.R. Radcliffe-Brown. Differently in France, an ethnological tradition grew in alignment with the work of Durkheim and his nephew Marcel Mauss and the avant-garde cultural movements exemplified by Marcel Griaule and Michel Leiris. However, despite thematic and analytical differences across the discipline, perspectives on culture, for much of the twentieth century, retained a view outwards to those under anthropological scrutiny, with little room for self-inspection or disciplinary reflexivity. Attempts to re-engage the concept 'culture' did not materialize until the sociologist Talcott Parsons forced anthropology to do so.

Parsons' project was to build upon the legacy of Durkheim and Weber to explain the objective consequences of human action and the norms and values that underpinned it (see Chapter 2). Doing so meant enlisting a three-part team of contributors: sociologists to study the social system, psychologists to study the role of personality and the individual, and anthropologists to study culture (as distinct from both the social system and the personalities that make it up). Parsons' newly established multidisciplinary Department of Social Relations at Harvard in 1946 embodied this division of labour. According to Parsons, anthropology had not yet established agreement on the culture concept: 'Only by some such definition of its scope can anthropology become an analytical empirical science which is independent both of sociology and of psychology' (Parsons in Kuper, 1999: 54) (Table 1.7). The challenge to pin down the culture concept demanded a response from the two leading anthropologists in the US at the time: Clyde Kluckhohn at Harvard and Alfred Kroeber at Berkeley. Together they set about a major review of anthropological theories, concepts and definitions. Working with 164 working conceptions of culture, in 1952 they produced the first formal definition of culture since Tylor in 1891 (Table 1.8).

For Kroeber and Kluckhohn, culture had to be treated as an integrated and structured whole, made up of connected parts. Tylor previously had included too many inventoried elements, with little to distinguish between culture and social organization. The idea was to narrow down the definition and to explicitly distinguish culture from society. Culture would, as a result, be observed directly in symbolic content, outward public expressions and embodiments that link together and characterize an integrated cultural system. Symbolism thus became central to the modern conception of culture and the development of cultural anthropology as a part of a distinctively North American discourse. This shift had an enduring influence on the young Clifford Geertz, a PhD graduate from the Department of Social Relations. Greatly influenced by Parsons, Weber, Ryle, Schutz and Wittgenstein, Geertz wanted to show how the symbolic meanings attributed to human actions could be read in a similar fashion to texts. His fieldwork in Indonesia and Morocco also produced a different context for study (Geertz, 1968). As societies caught in the transition from colonial rule to independence, they afforded a move beyond the heretofore static orientation to culture and an opportunity to read the symbolic role of ritual within the context of social change. Geertz produced a series of consistent definitions of culture over the course of his life, laying the basis for what would be understood as symbolic anthropology (Table 1.9). Culture, understood in terms of a web of observable symbols, was in the world and public, provided we knew where and, more importantly, *how* to look. However, despite Geertz's substantial contribution, for the better part of the twentieth century, studies of culture were still characterized by the well-established tensions between evolutionism and relativism, universalism and particularism, in addition to Claude Lévi-Strauss's innovation 'structuralism' – the idea that culture was generated by an ordering matrix, or grammar, encompassing structural rules and underlying patterns (Lévi-Strauss, 1963) (Table 1.10). Structuralism sought to demonstrate how classificatory systems are integral to social life and how cultural phenomena, such as totemism, rituals, kinship and so on, are products or reflections of contrasting categories. Outside of French intellectual inquiry, structuralism had a major impact on British anthropologists, most notably in the work of Edmund Leach, Mary Douglas, Victor Turner and Stanley Tambiah.

The status of these paradigms – symbolic anthropology, neo-evolutionism and structuralism, what Sherry Ortner (1984: 128) refers to as the 'theoretical bricoleur's kit', came under increasing scrutiny from the 1960s onwards. Assailed by a catalogue of real-world events, the processes of globalization, new identity politics, in addition to the rise in importance of the intellectual arenas of linguistics, literary theory, psychoanalysis, semiotics, political economy and subaltern studies, the discipline of anthropology became increasingly subject to critique. The critiques were both internal, levelled by a new generation of fieldworkers (Asad, 1973; Ortner, 1984; Rosaldo, 1989), and came from without, particularly from neo-Marxist sociologists, who challenged the discipline's weak attention to history and power, particularly colonial power. The culture concept was yet again undermined by the intensified movement of people, capital, things and ideas. It was repositioned for deconstruction and reconstruction in new disciplinary terms, particularly by the emerging field of cultural studies. Anthropology, according to Eric Wolf (1980), was coming apart because it was losing its grip on its most valued *raison d'être* – the explication of culture.

Despite the turmoil within the discipline, a consolidated reassessment of the culture concept did not appear until the publication of *Writing Culture* in 1986 (Clifford and Marcus, 1986) (Table 1.11). This marked a turning point, as the principal object of the publication was a critique of the ethnographic practice of writing and its capacity to fashion its object of interest: culture. *Writing Culture* was an explicit challenge to the authoritative position of the scientific observer. There could be no view from nowhere, no privileged perspectives, no neutral voiceover. The ethnographer was to be understood as actor, rather than auditor, and culture, rather than determining forms of sociality, was a collaborative product: an outcome of social practice in which the anthropologist was also implicated. This reflected a major turn for many anthropologists and focused attention on a new research agenda: an 'anthropology of the contemporary', as an emergent and contingent force of history (Rabinow, 2007) (Table 1.12).

The constitution of cultural reality and claims to truth as social practices, in and of themselves, was, in fact, not entirely new. It took its lead from Wittgensteinian philosophy and phenomenology and had been exemplified in sociological approaches such as ethnomethodology and the expanding domain of science and technology studies, similarly dependent on ethnographic forms of inquiry and the elucidation of cultural concerns. The attention to culture as the product of social practices moved this concept onwards – not only as a resource in and of anthropology to make sense of the world, but also as a resource employed by other social actors to construct and draw attention to those social differences at stake for them. This next section provides an example of one such domain – biomedicine – where culture is routinely invoked in the act of naming and problematizing difference.

Biomedicine: troubles in the invocation of culture

Biomedicine is an arena where invocations of culture can teach us much about the nature of its underlying assumptions as well as its enduring status as 'a trans-historical, transcultural model of reality' (Treichler, 1999: 119), that is, as an institutional arena that stands outside of culture's contaminating influences. The various distinctions that are, thereby, inferred by the natural-scientific/technical and the social-scientific/cultural dyad have been conventionally exercised through dualistic forms of reasoning captured by mind–body, health–illness distinctions. Critiques that have focused their efforts on deconstructing such divisions are well rehearsed across sociology and anthropology. Bruno Latour and Steve Woolgar's (1986) seminal ethnography *Laboratory Life*, for one, demonstrates that scientific knowledge and its representations do not stand outside of the contexts and practices within which they are embedded, and show the work of science to be an important cultural domain in its own right, with biology and medicine reconceived as complex cultural representations (Mulkay, 1979). However, conceptualizing culture thus from without cannot be said to have had much success in changing biomedicine's own epistemological paradigm, and culture largely persists as something that it encounters rather than that out of which it is made.

In teasing out the concept of culture through a focus on HIV/AIDS-related interventions, Julie Taylor (2007) provides a critical overview of the concept and its place at the intersections between medical anthropology, public health and epidemiology. In so doing, she draws attention to the often compromised status of anthropology as a discipline when attempting to engage with more authoritative and established forms of reasoning. Taylor challenges a propensity within biomedicine to view culture as a force that *acts* on disease, assuming it to be a 'cause' of or indeed a 'solution' to health-related problems. She argues that in an attempt to carve out a space within the healthcare arena, applied anthropologists, in particular, have often been at pains to show the positive potential of culture to assist medical interventions. In this regard, we can refer to the sizeable work that focuses on the significance and acquisition of 'cultural competence', as well as work that critically reflects upon it.[4] Taylor's broader point, however, is that mobilization of the concept – as cause or solution – leaves the concept itself unexamined and essentialized by being linked to more generalized cultural traits. One area where we see culture repeatedly positioned as a cause for concern is in the domain of transplant medicine and in the various anthropological and ethnographic analyses conducted in response to it. The following section takes up these issues by reference to empirical studies.

Organ transplantation and the cultural encounter

The demand for transplantable organs currently exceeds supply in most countries. It is a problem regularly couched in crisis terms – a problem that could be considered paradoxically of transplant medicine's own design (Sharp, 2006), but where responsibility is, in fact, often levelled at the idea of a poorly or partially participating public (Lock, 2002).

Margaret Lock's detailed examination of brain-death controversies and their impact on the development of deceased organ transplantation in North America and Japan provides a cross-cultural lens on the problematization of culture. Transplant medicine in Japan has been characterized by a resistance to the institutionalization of brain-death criteria among both the Japanese medical community and the public. Efforts to understand why have focused attention on religious beliefs and the country's deep-rooted cultural traditions. According to Lock: 'Of course, these values and behaviors can be conveniently glossed as cultural, and it is to such phenomena that Japanese refer when they argue that culture is implicated in the brain-death problem' (Lock, 2002: 8). However, for Lock, cultural explanations do not infer causality, nor do they provide us with a self-evident description of what the issues are. Instead, we need to tease out what exactly is being inferred when culture is invoked in these instances. In distinguishing between the USA and Japan, she shows how culture is used to isolate the practices of one group in anachronistic or deficit terms, as has been the case with the Japanese. Instead of examining why the Japanese have been resistant to the implementation of brain-death criteria until very recently, she reverses the question to ask, 'why did we in the "West" accept the remaking of death by medical professionals with so little public discussion?' (Lock, 2002: 4). By explicating culture in its specificities, we gain insight into the production of normative-anti-normative positions in medicine as well as an understanding of the broader political ends that are implicated in the complex struggle to advance or curtail the reach of transplant medicine in different settings.

Similar concerns are brought to the fore in Sherine Hamdy's (2012) analysis of transplant medicine in Egypt. In this context, Hamdy challenges the ways in which Islam, as an authoritative national institution, is drawn on to account for the resistances towards deceased organ donation. She shows that the cultural and ethical norms bound up with religious belief and practice do not necessarily map onto forms of decision-making in the provision or allocation of organs; nor can they account for the structural inequalities that have, as a result, shaped the profoundly unequal access to technologized medicine in Egypt. In a country marred by disparity, corruption and state failures, Hamdy's project is to recast the more conventional turn to bioethical and cultural considerations when explaining transplant medicine's failures to engage its publics, or indeed its practitioners, to one that emphasizes the role of the political economy in which transplant medicine is firmly embedded. Similar to Lock, she reverses what is often assumed as the logical question to ask when transplant medicine struggles for traction. As she puts it:

> Thus rather than simply asking why 'Egyptian culture' or 'Islam' operates as a constraint on potential biotechnical solutions, I ask instead why these technologies in fact do not appear to provide solutions to many in Egypt under their present circumstances.
>
> (Hamdy, 2012: 15)

For both Lock and Hamdy, difficulties in implementing biotechnologies such as organ transplantation cannot easily be reduced to a notion of culture that lies outside of it and acts upon it. That particular view of culture masks a whole range of other forces that are also cultural in character: institutional practices, the discursive representations of technology and the politics of access and allocation of healthcare resources. However, the lesson, in this particular case, is not to get caught up in working out what culture is and how it ought to be applied, but to show how it emerges as the product of exclusionary technologies – those used to mark out zones of difference. By way of a final illustration, I draw on an empirical example from work I have conducted with a colleague in the UK: its focus is to make visible the cultural work bound up with the production of racial categorizations in the context of organ donation and allocation in the UK (Kierans and Cooper, 2011).

In the UK, efforts to increase the supply of organs has led to a problematization of the comparatively low organ donation rates attributed to Britain's black and Asian populations, often grouped as 'BME' (black and minority ethnic) communities, in this case, people from African Caribbean and South Asian backgrounds. People within this category are commonly described as three to four times more likely than the white British population to develop end-stage kidney disease (Randhawa, 2010). They constitute approximately 28 per cent of the kidney transplant waiting list, but only 4 per cent of deceased organ donors (NHSBT, 2011). Because transplant practices in the UK favour organ-sharing within ethnic groupings due to matching human leukocyte antigens (HLAs) or blood and tissue matching, this translates into longer waits for suitable organs, and disparities in access to organ transplantation (Rudge et al., 2007).

This problem of inequality has driven healthcare researchers to focus attention on why 'BME' groups donate less, often translated as research into elucidating 'cultural barriers' – a term used loosely to include anything from religious beliefs to mortuary practices to issues of language and problems of assimilation (see Kierans and Cooper, 2011, for full discussion). While we can agree that reducing culture to random traits only serves to homogenize large groups of loosely connected individuals, these assumptions are, nevertheless, built into the development of health promotion and health policy. Indeed, they have led to a range of initiatives and media campaigns specifically aimed at members of 'black' and 'South Asian' 'communities'

(a) (b)

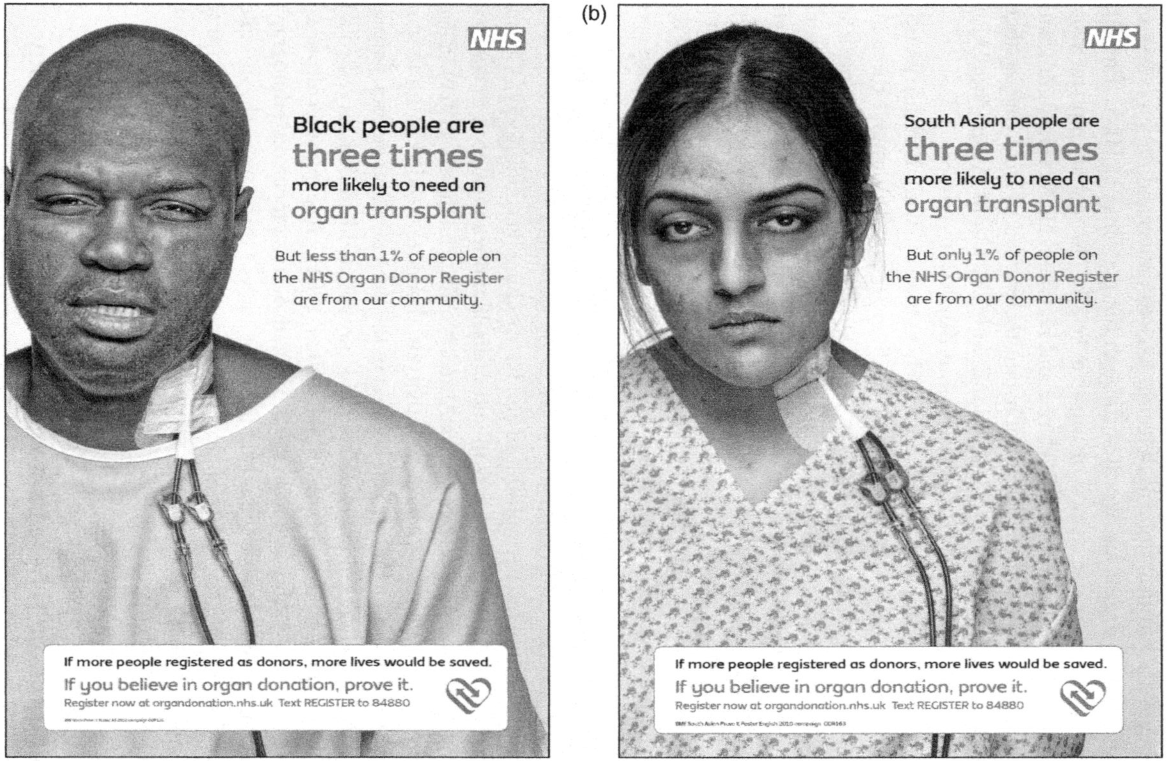

FIGURE 1.1 AND 1.2 Publicity for NHSBT's 'Prove it' campaign targeted to promote organ donation among 'minority ethnic groups' in the UK in 2009. Reprinted with permission of Wyatt-Clarke & Jones.

characterizing organ donation as a moral imperative, a collective responsibility *of* and *for* biologically and culturally distinct and distinguishable communities (see Figures 1.1 and 1.2).

To understand why race has emerged as a problem for organ donation, we need to look beyond a statistical story of donation rates to understand the processes and practices by which organs are allocated through the matching of HLAs. Ensuring a close match reduces the chance of organ rejection. Doctors attempt to match six different types of HLAs between donor and recipient. HLAs vary significantly across humans; however, their distributions are represented in medicine as aligning to established racial/ethnic classifications, with 'black' and 'Asian' populations described as having different HLA distributions than 'white' groups.

There is a bigger problem. HLAs vary widely in humans, with their distributions broadly owing to the geographic origins of different populations and thousands of years of population mixing (Marsh et al., 2000). However, in the transplant literature, what are highly complex variations are typically described in analytically unstable racial terms (Gordon, 2002). The criteria, therefore, used to determine who can be matched with whom are based on treating social and cultural membership as proxies for genetic makeup. Through attempts to accommodate 'rare' HLA types, transplant medicine has thus fallen back on the same classificatory schemas that were implicated in the creation of the inequalities health promotion initiatives were designed to address.

This example shows us that if we want to understand why culture has been invoked, we need to understand the matrices of social and institutional practice within which culture has been produced and has meaning (Hacking, 1999). Culture, therefore, has no explanatory power in and of itself and recourse to it as a way of explaining health outcomes exemplifies Alfred North Whitehead's (1929) 'fallacy of misplaced concreteness'. Critical sensitivity is, therefore, needed to understand the varied ways in which culture can be used in the exercise of biopolitics, particularly in situations where culturally defined 'risk' groups are identified, surveilled and regulated in relation to their health (Abu-Lughod, 1991).[5] To explicate culture as a mode of inquiry, Lila Abu-Lughod (1991: 149) advocates a focus on 'ethnographies of the particular' – ways of fostering forms of analysis that convey the complex macro- and micro-processes and practices that underpin culture's use and construction. The final section considers some methodological concerns for preserving culture as a mode of inquiry.

Assuming culture is here to stay: implications for methodology

To work with culture as the outcome of social processes and practices – i.e., to focus on culture as an end-point, a naming of difference, a term of invocation drawn on by various social actors in the course of social practice – is one way (among others) of working with the concept. This is what is suggested by the examples above. Doing so turns attention away from thinking about culture as an analytical tool used by anthropologists in an effort to explain the lives of others, to examining how it functions – as a resource put to work by our informants in the course of their everyday lives, or indeed mobilized within the 'marketplace of global discourse' referred to by Agar earlier in the chapter. For Agar, the work of culture involves the 'naming of a translation' or the identification of 'rich points' (Agar, 2006: 2). He suggests that culture emerges as a matter of concern when differences appear with reference to a newcomer or an outsider. The shape that culture takes depends on what he refers to as the 'of whom/for whom boundary'. Culture, as a result,

> isn't a property of *them*, nor is it a property of *us*. It is an artificial construction built to enable translation *between* them and us, *between* source and target. It is *intersubjective*, as the jargon says. It needs to be elaborate enough to get the job done and no more elaborate than that. If source and target are already similar in meanings and contexts, it will take less *culture* to do the job than if source and target are far apart. The translation we build *is* the culture we describe. Culture is relational. There is no *culture* of X, only a culture *of* X *for* Y. How much and what needs to go into that cultural description depends on which X and which Y define the boundary. In that way at least, culture is the same as translation.
>
> (Agar, 2006: 6, emphasis in original)

The job of the anthropologist is to take this translation and then trace back to the multiple, disparate, frequently idiosyncratic and happenstance ways that work to generate such rich points, those that in time become stabilized and naturalized as forms of understanding. Seeing culture in this way also means that we revisit the originally bounded and traditional anthropological subject – *the* Navajo, Yoruba or Trobriand Islander – as if they in their givenness ever represented a logical starting point for anthropological analysis, a means by which to neatly carve out the space of self and other, home and abroad, familiar and exotic, all of which had for so long anchored the anthropological imagination. In their essay 'Beyond "culture": space, identity and the politics of difference', Akhil Gupta and James Ferguson advocate that cultural groups – past and present – be re-read as outcomes of historical and social processes, endpoints, rather than departure points, in the production of difference. They suggest it is 'the premise of discontinuity' that ought to form 'the starting point from which to theorize contact, conflict, and contradiction between cultures and societies' (Gupta and Ferguson, 1992: 6).

Proceeding thus has provided a methodological starting point for many scholars in attempting to gain purchase on a world underpinned by the intensified movement of people, capital, things and ideas – one characterized by 'complex, overlapping and disjunctive orders' (Appadurai, 1990: 296) where the stability of group identity is perennially in question, as we have seen in the previous section with regard to 'BME' organ donors. It marks a distinct departure from the idea of culture as an object to be described and inventoried as Tylor once thought. Such 'traditional' orientations to differences, in the view of Donna Haraway (1991), have been cannibalized, giving over to more hybridized, mutable forms.

The methodological and ethnographic shift implied here is one that Ian Hacking advocates as increasingly bound up with elucidating and identifying the 'engines of discovery': those devices that produce, categorize, differentiate and 'make up' people, which turn groups into entities that were not there before (Hacking, 2006).[6] Statistics, medicine and biology are all significant engines of discovery – so too is a discipline such as anthropology, with its capacity to produce categories of analysis that name what is perceived a cultural difference. However, in placing our own engines of discovery under scrutiny, as the reflexive turn in anthropology has done, we can no longer assume the authoritative position of interlocutors for those who *cannot speak for themselves*. Attempts to do so, as James Clifford suggests, involve simplification and exclusion and lead to the construction of self–other relationships that imply the imposition or negotiation of a power relationship (Clifford, 1988).

Whether the culture concept retains its vitality for anthropology remains to be seen. For many anthropologists, however, it remains an important way to speak about or mark out differences, differences that have moral and political implications. And some of those implications arise precisely due to the ways in which culture is invoked in the context of social, political and economic affairs, or stabilized as part of an invisible, hegemonic background to everyday life. As Antonio Gramsci would have it, when culture becomes hegemonic, part of common-sense understandings, it masks a politics that is harder to notice, much less resist (Hoare and Nowell-Smith, 1971). To see culture then as the explicit naming of difference can provide a much-needed analytical lens on the processes of exclusion, stratification, identity formation, inequality, power and so on. Rather than employ the concept themselves, then, the task for many anthropologists is to examine how the concept is employed by others, particularly in debates – contemporary and historical – on the boundaries of civilizations, cultures, classes, races, genders, genes and the bodies and selves of others. Whatever way we approach difference, however, it remains clear that problematizing culture is a problematic exercise and it is there that anthropology's value may very well still lie.

Conclusion

In conclusion, let us return to Agar, who suggests: 'For now let's continue with culture, continue to redefine the concept so that we can say "culture means this", even if we know what we say hasn't the chance of the proverbial snowball in hell of ever influencing popular uses of the term' (Agar, 2006: 5). Perhaps our capacity to influence its usage is beside the point. What we can, however, show are the many different ways in which culture comes to matter for others, as well as the problematic politics that lie within it. The invocation of culture helps us to identify 'rich points': a way of mapping a translation of difference, itself the product of practices that require interrogation. It is this mapping that maintains an important role for the anthropologist-ethnographer – as interlocutor in the spaces where culture comes to be made and remade.

Notes

1 *Verstehen* is a German term associated with the sociologist Max Weber and his emphasis on interpretivism (see Chapter 2). Its meaning is to understand, perceive, know and comprehend the nature and significance of a phenomenon. Weber used the term to refer to the social scientist's attempt to understand both the intention and the context of human action.
2 For example, in his book *The Fateful Hoaxing of Margaret Mead*, the anthropologist Derek Freeman (1999) argues that Mead was deceived by mischievous informants and that the picture she painted of Samoan adolescence was largely inaccurate.
3 It's important to mention that for Benedict and many of her contemporaries who were embedded in the war effort (World War II), orientations to culture were shaped not simply by distinctions between nations but also by efforts to marshal those distinctions and render them intelligible for military purposes. *The Chrysanthemum and the Sword*, Benedict's monograph on culture and personality in Japan, grew out of wartime research she did for the American State Department and Office of War Information (Fukui, 1999).
4 For an overview of work in this area, see for example Gershon and Taylor's (2008) 'Culture in the spaces of no culture' and Willen and Carpenter-Song's (2013) 'Cultural competence in action: multidisciplinary perspectives on four case studies'.
5 While medical approaches to working with the culture concept are vulnerable to the assumption that culture-bearers are those that exist *outside* of the institutional domain of medicine, it is important not to oversimplify practices in health and medicine either and to appreciate that many working in those domains have also actively engaged in much reflection and revision of the concept (see Kirmayer, 2012).
6 For further discussion in relation to the body, see Chapter 7.

References

Abu-Lughod, L. (1991) Writing against culture. In R.G. Fox (ed.), *Recapturing Anthropology: Working in the Present*. Santa Fe, NM: School of American Research Press, 137–162.

Agar, M. (2006) Culture: Can you take it anywhere? *International Journal of Qualitative Methods*, 5(2): 1–12.

Appadurai, A. (1990) Disjuncture and difference in the global cultural economy. In M. Featherstone (ed.), *Global Culture: Nationalism, Globalization and Modernity*. London: Sage, 295–310.

Asad, T (ed.) (1973) *Anthropology and the Colonial Encounter*. Ithaca: London.

Benedict, R. (1934) *Patterns of Culture*. New York: Houghton Mifflin.

Boas, F. (1911) *The Mind of Primitive Man*. New York: The MacMillan Company.

Bourdieu, P. (1984) *Distinctions: A Social Critique of the Judgement of Taste*. Cambridge, MA: Harvard University Press.

Clifford, J. (1988) *The Predicament of Culture: Twentieth Century Ethnography, Literature and Art*. Cambridge, MA: Harvard University Press.

Clifford, J. and Marcus, G. (eds.) (1986) *Writing Culture: the Politics and Poetics of Ethnography*. Berkeley, CA: University of California Press.

Elias, N. (1978 [1939]) *The Civilizing Process: The History of Manners*, Vol. 1. Translated by E. Jephcott. Oxford: Blackwell.
Frankenberg, R. (1995) Learning from AIDS: the future of anthropology. In A.S. Ahmed and C. N. Shore (eds.), *The Future of Anthropology: Its Relevance to the Contemporary World*. London: Athlone Press, 11–33.
Freeman, D. (1999) *The Fateful Hoaxing of Margaret Mead*. New York: Basic Books.
Fukui, N. (1999) Background research for *The Chrysanthemum and the Sword*. *Dialectical Anthropology*, 24(2): 173–180.
Gaughan, M.I. and Lutzeier, P.R. (2007) *German Art 1907–1937: Modernism and Modernisation*, German Linguistic and Cultural Studies, Vol. 19. Oxford: Peter Lang.
Geertz, C. (1968) *Islam Observed: Religious Development in Morocco and Indonesia*. Chicago, IL: University of Chicago Press.
Geertz, C. (1973) *The Interpretation of Cultures*. New York: Basic Books.
Gershon, I. and Taylor, J. (2008) Culture in the spaces of no culture. *American Anthropologist*, 110(4): 417–421.
Gordon, E. (2002) What 'race' cannot tell us about access to kidney transplantation. *Cambridge Quarterly of Healthcare Ethics*, 11(2): 134–141.
Greenfield, S. (2001) Nature/nurture and the anthropology of Franz Boas and Margaret Mead as an agenda for revolutionary politics. *Horizontes Antropológicos*, 7(16): 35–52.
Grimshaw, A. and Hart, K. (1993) *Anthropology and the Crisis of Intellectuals*. Cambridge, MA: Prickly Pear Press.
Gupta, A. and Ferguson, J. (1992) Beyond 'culture': space, identity and the politics of difference. *Cultural Anthropology*, 7(1): 6–23.
Hacking, I. (1999) *The Social Construction of What?* Cambridge, MA: Harvard University Press.
Hacking, I. (2006) Making up people. *London Review of Books*, 28(16): 23–26.
Hamdy, S. (2012) *Our Bodies Belong to God: Organ Transplants, Islam and the Struggle for Human Dignity in Egypt*. Berkeley, CA: University of California Press.
Haraway, D. (1991) *Simians, Cyborgs and Women: The Reinvention of Nature*. New York: Routledge.
Harris, M. (1968) *The Rise of Anthropological Theory: A History of Theories of Culture*. New York: Thomas Y. Cromwell Co.
Hoare, Q. and Nowell-Smith, G. (eds.) (1971) *Selections from the Prison Notebooks of Antonio Gramsci*. London: Lawrence & Wishart Ltd.
Kierans, C. and Cooper, J. (2011) Organ donation, genetics, race and culture: the making of a medical problem. *Anthropology Today*, 27(6): 21–25.
Kirmayer, L. (2012). Rethinking cultural competence. *Transcultural Psychiatry*, 49(2): 149–164.
Kroeber, A. L. and Kluckhohn, C. (1952) Culture: a critical review of concepts and definitions. *Papers of the Peabody Museum of Archaeology and Ethnology*, Vol. XLVII, No. 1. Cambridge, MA: Harvard University.
Kuper, A. (1999) *Culture: the Anthropologists' Account*. Cambridge, MA: Harvard University Press.
Latour, B. and Woolgar, S. (1986) *Laboratory Life: the Construction of Scientific Facts*. Princeton, NJ: Princeton University Press.
Lévi-Strauss, C. (1963) *Structural Anthropology*. New York: Basic Books.
Lévi-Strauss, C (1969 [1949]) *The Elementary Structures of Kinship*. Translated by J. Bell. Boston, MA: Beacon Press.
Lock, M. (2002) *Twice Dead: Organ Transplants and the Reinvention of Death*. Berkeley, CA: University of California Press.
Malinowski, B. (1922) *Argonauts of the Western Pacific*. London: Routledge and Kegan Paul.
Malinowski, B. (1927) *Sex and Repression in Savage Society*. London: Kegan Paul, Trench Trubner and Co.

Malinowski, B. (1931) Culture. In E.R.A. Seligman (ed.), *Encyclopedia of the Social Sciences, Vol. 4*. New York: Macmillan, 621–646.
Marsh, S.G.E., Parham, P. and Barber, L.D. (2000) *The HLA Facts Book*. San Diego, CA: Academic Press.
Mead, M. (1928) *Coming of Age in Samoa*. New York: HarperCollins.
Mead, M. (1937) *Cooperation and Competition Among Primitive People*. New York: McGraw-Hill.
Mulkay, M. (1979) *Science and the Sociology of Knowledge*, London: Boston: G. Allen & Unwin.
NHSBT (2011) Transplant activity in the UK. *Activity Report 2010/11*. Available at: https://nhsbtmediaservices.blob.core.windows.net/organ-donation-assets/pdfs/activity_report_2010_11.pdf.
North Whitehead, A. (1929) *Process and Reality*. New York: Macmillan.
Ortner, S. (1984) Theory in anthropology since the sixties. *Comparative Studies in Society and History*, 26(1): 126–166.
Parsons, T. (1951) *The Social System*. London: Routledge and Kegan Paul Ltd.
Porter, R. (2001) *The Enlightenment*. Basingstoke: Palgrave Macmillan.
Rabinow, P. (1986) Representations as social facts: modernity and post-modernity in anthropology. In J. Clifford and G. Marcus (eds.), *Writing Culture: The Politics and Poetics of Ethnography*. Berkeley: University of California Press, 234–261.
Rabinow, P. (2007) *Marking Time: On the Anthropology of the Contemporary*. Princeton, NJ: Princeton University Press.
Radcliffe-Brown, A.R. (1922) *The Andaman Islanders: A Study in Social Anthropology*. Cambridge: Cambridge University Press.
Radcliffe-Brown, A.R. (1940) On social structure. *The Journal of the Royal Anthropological Institute of Great Britain and Ireland*, 70(1): 1–12.
Randhawa, G. (2010) Renal health disparities in the United Kingdom: a focus on ethnicity. *Seminars in Nephrology*, 30: 8–11.
Rosaldo, R. (1989) *Culture and Truth: the Remaking of Social Analysis*. Boston: Beacon Press.
Rudge, C., Johnson, R.J., Fuggle, S.V. and Forsythe, J.L.R. (2007) Renal transplantation in the United Kingdom for patients from ethnic minorities. *Transplantation*, 83(9): 1169–1173.
Sapir, E. (1921) *Language: An Introduction to the Study of Speech*. New York: Harcourt, Brace and Company.
Sharp, L. (2006) *Strange Harvest: Organ Transplants, Denatured Bodies, and the Transformed Self*. Berkeley, CA: University of California Press.
Stocking, G.W. (1966) Franz Boas and the culture concept in historical perspective. *American Anthropologist*, 68(4): 867–882.
Stocking, G.W. (1974) *The Shaping of American Anthropology, 1883–1911: A Franz Boas Reader*. New York: Basic Books.
Taylor, J. (2007) Assisting or compromising intervention? The concept of 'culture' in biomedical and social research on HIV/AIDS. *Social Science and Medicine*, 64(4): 965–975.
Treichler, P. (1999) *How to Have Theory in an Epidemic: Cultural Chronicles of AIDS*. Durham, NC: Duke University Press.
Tylor, E.B. ([1958] 1871) *Primitive Culture*. London: John Murray.
Willen, S. and Carpenter-Song, E. (2013) Cultural competence in action: multi-disciplinary perspectives on four case studies. *Culture, Medicine and Psychiatry*, 37(2): 241–397.
Wolf, E. (1980) They divide and subdivide and call it anthropology. *New York Times*, 30 November: E9.

2

SOCIETY

Carol Kingdon

> There exists a wealth of social phenomena which occur over the whole of society, but which assume various forms according to regions, occupations, religious faiths, etc. Such are, for instance, crime, suicide, birth. From the diversity of these particular environments there result, for each of these new orders of facts, new series of variations beyond those which historical evolution has produced.
>
> Émile Durkheim, *The Rules of the Sociological Method*

Introduction

Society, like culture, is a contested concept. While no longer the preserve of a single discipline (if indeed it ever was), sociology remains synonymous with society as a central concern (Frisby and Sayer, 1986). This is despite, if not because of, the lack of consensus surrounding its defining characteristics. As Raymond Williams suggests: 'society is now clear in two main senses: as our most general term for the body of institutions and relationships within which a relatively large group of people live: and as our most abstract term for the condition in which such institutions and relationships are formed' (cited in Elliot and Turner, 2012: 3). Sociology as a discipline was born of the twin processes of intellectual crisis brought about by the Enlightenment, and economic and social change stemming from the Industrial Revolution. The development of social theories of individualization, neoliberalism, globalization and the communications revolution represent new concerns fuelling claims that society is now an outdated concept – a meaningless category for present-day existence (Beck and Beck-Gernsheim, 2002). It is significant, however, that while some sociologists have turned away from society as a conceptual resource, it has gained prominence elsewhere, such as in the particular (positivist) vision of the social advanced through 'social determinants' discourses in public health medicine.

This chapter traces the various trajectories taken by society as a concept, asserting its foundational place within sociology as a discipline.[1] It argues for a return to the concept of society (in all its guises) to advance cross-disciplinary agendas for health – an arena where its mutability may be considered a strength and a means of opening up multiple lines of enquiry, both old and new. Among others, the chapter draws from the writings of Émile Durkheim at the end of the nineteenth century, whose work offers an anchor point for the chapter as a whole. Questions of why society is important, how it is held together, made and remade, and what the relationship is between the individual and society are highlighted as enduring concerns for social science scholars grappling with the complexity of modernity and social change. These concerns coalesce with the kinds of questions health professionals more commonly ask about the social patterning of health inequalities, the meanings and actions of individuals, and how medicine, technology and healthcare impact the contemporary experience of health and illness, with stillbirth used as a case study to tease out the present-day utility of society as a conceptual resource.

This chapter offers social scientists and health professionals an overview of the ways in which society has been conceptualized and how we might utilize the concept moving forward. In so doing, the chapter aims to achieve three things. First, it demonstrates how society has been taken up by social scientists, the relationships between these positions, and their promise. Second, it shows how a particular vision of the social has been employed in the field of public health, which is both partial and problematic. Third and finally, it highlights the promise of the concept when taken as multiple. As with the preceding discussion of culture, this chapter makes no claim to be comprehensive, but instead maps key shifts in the concept's career. Definitions in support of society as a concept can be found in Table 2.

Where to start: the problem of society and its promise

Most simply, the term 'society' refers to a bounded unit (Hughes et al., 2003). Human life is impossible in isolation. Our food chain, where we sleep, the work we do, how we communicate and the institutions that govern the ways that we live together (family, education, medicine) are aspects of the social that are encapsulated in the term 'society'. Thus, what is most interesting about society is *how* people live together and with what consequences. As the sociologist Charles Wright Mills (1959) highlighted more than 50 years ago (Table 2.1):

> We have come to know that every individual lives, from one generation to the next, in some society: that he lives out a biography, and that he lives it out within some historical sequence. By the fact of his living he contributes, however minutely, to the shaping of this society and to the course of its history, even as he is made by society and its historical push and shove. The

TABLE 2 Definitions of society

2.1 Charles Wright Mills (1959: 3)	Neither the life of an individual nor the history of a society can be understood without understanding both.
2.2 Èmile Durkheim (1982 [1895]: 248)	Human societies present a new phenomenon of a special nature, which consists in the fact that certain ways of acting are imposed, or at least suggested *from outside* the individual and are added on to his own nature.
2.3 Herbert Spencer (1897 [1897]: 447–448)	The permanent relations among the parts of a society are analogous to the permanent relations among the parts of a living body.
2.4 Auguste Comte (Comte and Martineau (2009 [1853]: 511)	Some metaphysical speculation there has been about the existence of general laws of society; but their germs have never been brought to light, nor their application to the most common and interesting phenomena been exhibited; but the exposition made in this work leaves no doubt of the universal presence of the principle.
2.5 Ferdinand Tönnies (1963 [1887]: 161)	Society is only a transitional and superficial phenomenon.
2.6 Georg Simmel (1992 [1895]: 55)	Society exists where several individuals (for one another, with one another or against one another) enter into interaction.
2.7 Gabriel Tarde (2008 [1899]: 35)	I explain collective resemblances of the whole by the massing together of minute elementary acts – greater by the lesser and the whole by the part.
2.8 Max Weber (1978: 4)	The interpretive understanding of human social action.
2.9 Erving Goffman (1959: 35)	When the individual presents himself before others, his performance will tend to incorporate and exemplify the officially accredited values of the society.
2.10 Talcott Parsons (1966: 10)	The core of a society, as a system is the patterned normative order through which the life of a population is collectively organized.
2.11 Anthony Giddens (1984: 162)	'Society' has a useful double meaning – signifying a bounded system, and social association in general (p. 162).
2.12 Karl Marx (1988 [1848]: 55–56)	The history of all hitherto existing societies is the history of class struggles. [...] We find almost everywhere a complicated arrangement of society into various orders, a manifold graduation of social rank.
2.13 Niklas Luhmann (1997: 72)	Under modern conditions, the global system is a society, in which all internal boundaries can be contested and all solidarities shift.
2.14 Bruno Latour (2005: 2)	I believe it's necessary to scrutinise more thoroughly the exact content of what is 'assembled' under the umbrella of a society. This seems to me the only way to be faithful to the old duties of society, this science of the living together.

> sociological imagination enables us to grasp history and biography and the relations between the two within society. That is its task and its promise.
>
> (Wright Mills, 1959: 6)

Such an outwardly simple idea – i.e., what it means to live together – is one of the few threads from which a coherent story of society as a concept can begin to be woven. In sociology, there are a number of scholars who have grappled with society as a concept, who collectively show both the enormity of the task and the significance of choosing an appropriate point of entry (Campbell, 1981; Frisby and Sayer, 1986; Nisbet, 1993; Lemert, 1995; Outhwaite, 2006; Elliot and Turner, 2012). This is especially important as the term society has been mobilized to do many different things within (and without) sociology. Wright Mills' starting point was to navigate between 'the personal troubles of milieu' and 'the public issues of social structure' (1959: 8), a dichotomy that has simultaneously tasked and inspired sociologists since the discipline's inception because it is 'within that range the sociological imagination has its chance to make a difference in the quality of human life' (1959: 226).

Since the nineteenth century, establishing critiques of the social has become central to the sociological tradition. The sheer volume of theorizing within the discipline has been underpinned by the pull of the individual/society dichotomy, demanding a commitment to one side or the other. Yet it is such contests between different visions of the social that have continuously sparked the sociological imagination. Society as a concept originated from the need to account for the force of the urban and industrial explosion in nineteenth-century Europe that changed how people lived together in ways that transcended their everyday existence as individuals. The sociological imagination did more than chart these changes; it theorized them and in so doing founded the 'science of the living together' (Latour, 2005: 2).

Society *sui generis*: the making of society as a distinct object of concern

Durkheim's (1952 [1897]: 38) claim that 'there can be no sociology unless societies exist, and societies cannot exist if there are only individuals' is illustrative both of his lifelong project to establish sociology as a science, and the significance of his conception of society to achieving this (Table 2.2). His first major work, *The Division of Labour in Society* (Durkheim, 1960 [1893]), drew on earlier formulations of society developed by French and Scottish Enlightenment scholars, including Adam Smith. Smith had previously introduced the term 'division of labour' to political philosophy to account for the distribution of tasks among individuals in a group to ensure that economic and domestic roles are performed by different people for the collective maintenance of society (Morrison, 2006). Where Durkheim differs from Smith is in observing a distinction between a social and economic division of labour, with the former providing the basis of social bonds and the foundations of society as a unique entity. In Durkheim's words, the division of labour 'passes far beyond purely economic interests, for it consists in the establishment of a social and moral order *sui generis*' (Durkheim, 1960 [1893]: 61). Thus, Durkheim conceived of society both as an independent entity and a moral phenomenon, where 'the totality of beliefs and sentiments common to average citizens of the same society forms a determinate system which has its own life; one may call it the *collective* or *common conscience*' (1960 [1893]: 79, emphasis in original). This was a definitive break from the Enlightenment conception that society is nothing more than the sum of individuals (Hughes et al., 2003). Instead, Durkheim (1960 [1893]: 129) asserted 'there are in each of us two consciences: one which is common to our group in its entirety, which consequently is not ourself, but society living and acting within us; the other, on the contrary represents that in us which is personal and distinct, that which makes us individual'.

What are now commonly thought of in terms of our social roles (wife, mother, daughter, wage-earner, responsible citizen), norms (the assumption that being married is important or that children will follow a marriage) and values (moral codes that inform the former behaviours) were at the heart of Durkheim's propositions of a 'collective conscience' and his conception of solidarity as the mechanism of integration for cohesiveness between individuals and society. In attempting to distinguish between different types of social orders, Durkheim emphasized a fundamental distinction between mechanical and organic solidarity to be mapped onto traditional social systems, on the one hand, and modern societies, on the other. In doing so, he drew a clear contrast between the complex modern order, where diverse interests are the source from which individuals derive solidarity and cohesion, and pre-modern societies, where solidarity is characterized by homogeneity and conformity of the group.

In developing this approach to society, Durkheim directly challenged the notion of industrial solidarity in Herbert Spencer's *Principles of Sociology* (1874). As indicated in Chapter 1, in seeking to explain Victorian Britain's trading success in evolutionary terms, Spencer had argued that social progress emerges out of competitive struggles between social groupings, with social gains arising from the evolutionary development of individuals: coining the phrase 'survival of the fittest' before Charles Darwin (Lee and Newby, 1989). Both Spencer and his contemporary Auguste Comte were heavily influenced by the advances of biology at the time, as evident in what were to become sociology's opening definitions of society (Table 2.3 and 2.4). While all three (Comte, Spencer and Durkheim) sought to show how the lessons learned in the natural sciences could be applied to the social world to re-engineer and improve society, Durkheim (1960 [1893]) rejected Spencer's claim that the individual may be 'effectively emancipated from collective influence' in the shift from traditional to industrial society (with the advent of wage labour). He suggested instead that 'we are mistaking a transformation for a disappearance' (1960 [1893]: 204) on the grounds that a society in which each individual solely pursues his or her own interests would disintegrate very quickly (Giddens, 1971).

It was, however, Comte who first conceived of a science of society in *Cours de Philosophie Positive* (Comte and Martineau, 2009 [1853]), underpinned by a positivist methodology,[2] one that Durkheim adopted and adapted to further his claim of society *sui generis* – emphasizing the critical importance of the social as an entity in and of itself (Durkheim, 1960 [1893]). In so doing, it was Durkheim who established the social as a distinct object of concern. This is succinctly illustrated in the conclusion of *The Rules of the Sociological Method*, with his assertion that 'if we consider social facts[3] as things, it is as *social things*' (Durkheim, 1982 [1895]: 162, emphasis in original), a proposition best exemplified in his influential and enduring study of suicide (Durkheim, 1952 [1897]). Prior to Durkheim, suicide was viewed entirely as a personal act and psychological fact. Through his analysis of 26,000 suicide records from France, Italy and Prussia, Durkheim's study of suicide showed that the degree of social integration and regulation in society can impact the suicide rate – establishing suicide as a social fact. In other words, a phenomenon hitherto thought of as being fundamentally individual was thus seen to have a social dimension. What is more, his view of psychological and physiological outcomes as having a social dimension made visible for the first time categories of stratification in society by religious affiliation, occupation, gender and age. This set a precedent for studies of social stratification that take into account not only more traditional systems of class, but other social categories too, and the intersection between them. In summary, it may be said that Durkheim's development of the society concept was as an organic whole born out of structured relations.

Between individuals: social (inter)action, community and society

Contemporaneous to the development of society as structure, an entirely different conception of society was being conceived – as an aggregate of processes of individual action (Table 2.5–2.8). Ferdinand Tönnies' (1963 [1887]) *Community and Society* was published in the decade preceding Durkheim's major works. While both shared concerns with changes in the way society is held together as a consequence of the transition from traditional to modern formations, they fundamentally differed in their conception of society in relation to the individual. For Tönnies, society and community were concepts to be applied to the everyday realities of human life and experience, with society realized through relationships between individuals – a theory of society that was to shape Max Weber's later work detailing how individuals orient their actions in relation to social groupings.

Bruno Latour's (2005) reading of Gabriel Tarde identifies that he too conceived the collective resemblances of the whole by its parts (Table 2.7). Tarde's (2008 [1899]) formulation of society ran contrary to Durkheim's by disputing that social facts and evolutionary laws guide individual actions. Instead, Tarde used science as one example of the power of human actions originating in and from individuals. Other analysts identify Georg Simmel as the most significant challenger to the concept of society *sui generis*. Simmel sought advance for sociology in the study of forms of human interaction and processes of sociation (*vergesellschaftung*). For Simmel the question was less 'what is the defining object of study for sociology as a science?' and more 'how is society possible?' Simmel claimed, 'society is a unity because and in so far as all its individuals interact'. In direct opposition to Durkheim's position he wrote, 'society is not an entity fully enclosed within itself, an absolute entity, any more than is the human individual. Compared with the real interaction of the parts it is only secondary, only the result' (cited in Frisby and Sayer, 1986: 55). Thus, the tension Wright Mills (1959) identifies between society and the individual was brought into play.

Writing in *Economy and Society*, Weber did not directly challenge Durkheim, but his opposition to society as an object in itself could not be clearer when he wrote 'sociology is a science concerning itself with the interpretive understanding of human social action' (Weber, 1978: 4). Weber's theory of social action was to provide the foundations for the interpretative tradition in sociology through his concept of *verstehen* (see Chapter 1). To dichotomize Durkheim and Weber's positions is dangerously simplistic; nevertheless, in relation to Weber's social action theory it may be said that Durkheim favoured positivism, objectivity and structure (the view from outside), while Weber favoured interpretivism, subjectivity and the actions of individuals towards other individuals (the view from within) (Hughes et al., 2003). Weber was most interested in the meanings individuals ascribe to action or, in other words, with what purpose actions are embarked upon.

Writing much later, the American sociologist Erving Goffman provided one example of how society conceived as structure and society as social action were taken up to enable multi-dimensional understandings of the complexity of everyday lived realities. Goffman's (1959) *The Presentation of Self in Everyday Life* theorized how individuals act both (through the processes of impression management) to 'stage' performances in the pursuit of social integration *and* for the functioning of society (Table 2.9), developing this line of argument further in *Stigma: Notes on the Management of Spoiled Identity* (1963). Goffman's (1963) approach highlighted the disjuncture between an individual's virtual social identity and their actual social identity. In other words, he emphasized the socially constructed normative role expectations of an individual that must be presented to prevent the self being discredited, as opposed to the attributes an individual actually possesses that are considered to be stigmatizing in and by society. Efforts to incorporate both structural constraints and individual action in explanations of society were a characteristic feature of twentieth-century sociology, with 'society' viewed as both structure *and* that which connects individuals providing a different starting point for the 'science of the living together'.

The dualities of structure and the fracturing of the social

The American sociologist Talcott Parsons (see Chapter 1) worked to build on Durkheim and Weber so as to explain the objective consequences of human action and the norms and values that underpinned it within a distinctly functionalist perspective. Parsons' (1937, 1951) structural functionalism offered a way of understanding society as a bounded system of discrete but interrelated parts that function as an organic whole (Table 2.10). Parsons re-emphasized the importance of moral consensus and social cohesion, and, in doing so, transformed these principles into a new programme for the social sciences, which would incorporate many leading scholars in the field, such as the British sociologist Anthony Giddens and the French sociologist Pierre Bourdieu.

It was Parsons' voluminous writings on society that provided the starting point for Giddens to later reformulate understanding of social structures (Lemert, 1995). Giddens' structuration theory (indebted to both Durkheim and Parsons) seeks to overcome the classical dualism of the individual and society by claiming the duality of social structures themselves: 'The structural properties of social systems are both medium and outcome of the practices they recursively organize' (Giddens, 1984: 25). Thus, society is simultaneously social structure, individual agency and transformation. Albeit from a different starting point, Bourdieu also attended to the subjectivism and objectivism dichotomy (see also Chapter 7). Bourdieu's (1977) working of the concept of 'habitus' (as the interplay between structure and practice) achieves a similar move to Giddens' structuration theory in encapsulating how structure and action reproduce social life. According to Lemert (1995), writing on Bourdieu, habitus serves to simultaneously ground what Durkheim connected to consciousness and Weber recognized as neither a subjective attitude nor an objective rule of the modern world. In other words, '*habitus* is that habit of moral action whereby individuals know how to act in a certain manner either without inventing the action each time they act thusly *or* without being told by any one thing or another thing (least of all structured society) just how to act' (Lemert, 1995: 142, emphasis in original).

Parsons' structural functionalist conception of society dominated mid-twentieth-century sociology until the political and economic shifts and new social movements of the 1960s and 1970s sparked interest in the development of the society concept as something other than a system functioning in harmony.[4] Giddens' structuration theory and Bourdieu's sociology of associations represent two of the many attempts to challenge the dualisms of classical thought and reconceive structure as less constraining, but no less important, in society. Jean-François Lyotard's (1984 [1979]) *The Postmodern Condition: A Report on Knowledge*, on the other hand, specifically sought to understand the implications for society of the control of knowledge and information through the changing status of science and technology, contesting the continued relevance of structure altogether.

Lyotard too critiqued earlier formulations of the society concept as dualistic, but in relation to society as a functional whole (structural functionalism) or society as divided in two (Marxist-derived class-based theories[5]). Lyotard challenged these 'grand narratives' with their claims of universality as 'out of step with the most vital modes of postmodern knowledge', suggesting 'what is new in all of this is that the old poles of attraction represented by nation-states, parties, professions, institutions, and historical traditions are losing their attraction' (Lyotard, 1984 [1979]: 14). This form of post-society critique was to be further developed as the century came to a close and new technologies and knowledge acquisition spawned a new phase of globalization, leading to claims of 'the intensification of worldwide social relations which link distant localities in such a way that local happenings are shaped by events occurring many miles away and vice versa' (Giddens, 1990: 64).

As stated in the introduction, the last decades of the twentieth century and the first decades of the twenty-first century are routinely characterized as entailing an intensification of economic and social change. It has been suggested that more recent waves of globalization represent a fundamental challenge to the society concept on the grounds that the latter solidifies social phenomena (fixing structures within states and national boundaries), whereas the former affords fluidity and malleability across traditional borders and categories (Wallerstein, 1986). John Urry's (2000) *Sociology Beyond Societies* asserts that the apparent decline of the nation-state brings the continued relevance of the society concept into question as global flows (trade, migration, information, culture) increasingly shape everyday realities. While for Niklas Luhmann (Table 2.13), the heart of the matter is the choice between seeing the global system as a society or as 'a system of societies' (Outhwaite, 2006: 51). Moreover, for Luhmann (1997: 73) the assumption of a world society should be the starting point to 'investigate how and why this society tends to maintain or even to increase regional inequalities'.

Latour's *Reassembling the Social* offers yet another way to take up and scrutinize 'more thoroughly what is "assembled" under the umbrella of a society' (2005: 2), which advocates rather than beginning with society or other social aggregates, one should end with them. For Latour it is no longer (if it ever was) sufficient to take society or the social as an overarching explanation in and of itself (Table 2.14). The task is to trace associations (including between humans and non-humans) to enable the social to remain fluid and where new conceptions of collectives may be assembled, but not fixed. This is an approach to society – like that of Giddens (1984), Bourdieu (1977) and Luhmann (1997) – that recognizes its conceptual ambiguity, but does not reject it in its entirety.

Conceptualizing society through the 'social determinants of health'

Although sociology is characterized by an increasingly cautious engagement with the concept of society, one in which its transparency and utility have been repeatedly challenged, these internal debates have had little effect on its uptake outside of the discipline. The *Black Report* (Townsend and Davidson, 1992 [1980]) and *The Health Divide* (Whitehead, 1992 [1987]) provide an illustrative example of the endurance and potency of the society concept as taken up in the context of public health medicine. Using statistical data from a range of official sources, these two major UK reports found that most of the major and minor killers in British society affected the poorest classes more than the richest – at every stage of life from birth to adulthood and into old age. In their aftermath, the 'social determinants of health' framework gained considerable momentum in the field of public health, both in the UK and internationally (see Dahlgren and Whitehead, 1992; Marmot and Wilkinson, 2006; Raphael, 2011). Broadly speaking, it refers to the societal factors, and the unequal distribution of these factors, which contribute to both overall health and existing inequalities in health. Associated more explicitly with developments in public health epidemiology rather than sociology, 'the social' is taken to represent the conditions in which people are born, grow, live, work and age, with these circumstances shaped by the distribution of money, power and resources at global, national and local levels (Commission on Social Determinants of Health, 2008; WHO, 2014a).

It has been a major achievement of public health to make the problem of health inequality real and actionable, giving rise to the influential 'health equity through social change' model (Preda and Voigt, 2015) and other related attempts to address the social roots of ill health. Today, the weight of evidence that health inequalities are the product of social and environmental factors is unassailable – with a relationship between health and labour market disadvantage (through unemployment or lower socioeconomic group), as well as cigarette smoking and social disadvantage, and social support and health especially well-established (Schofield, 2007). But the social determinants of health approach (resonate of Durkheim's positivism) is not without its problems. Indeed, as Toni Schofield observes:

> the evidence presented demonstrates the existence of a relationship between a social condition(s) or factor(s) and a specific health problem but it rarely shows the *mechanisms* by which the social produces the problem. In the absence of evidence and explanation demonstrating *how* the social works in producing the problem, the recommended policy interventions devised to address the social dynamics are *speculative*.
>
> (Schofield, 2007: 108, emphasis in original)

Moreover, they often tend to be applied in ways that end up emphasizing the 'downstream' determinants of health, leading to approaches that are depoliticized and individualized, such as programmes focusing on lifestyle risk behaviours (Brassolotto et al., 2014). Thus, the rise of the social determinants of health framework has done little to dislodge the 'hidden reliance upon the framework of biomedical individualism' (Krieger, 1994: 887).

Judith Green's (2010) editorial on the World Health Organization's (WHO) Commission on Social Determinants of Health highlights the vast body of evidence documenting inequalities, and the utter lack of evidence of what works to reduce health inequity, which she attributes in part to how poorly health inequity is conceptualized. She also identifies the challenges that arise from ideological differences when policy begins to be implemented in real communities: 'then the consensus threatens to fracture, over which domains of health are prioritized, whose rights are being defended, or how we know whether "more health" is being achieved or not' (Green, 2010: 3). This is a line of argument that resonates with Latour's (2005) concerns about the premature fixing of the social, with the present period of globalization of Westernized medicine (its processes, polices and technologies) providing a particularly interesting lens on ways of thinking about and (re)configuring ideas of the social that move beyond determinist structural functionalist frameworks.

The next section uses stillbirth as a case study to demonstrate a number of different ways the concept of society may be taken up to advance understanding of the social patterning of health inequalities, the meanings and actions of individuals, and how medicine, technology and healthcare impact the contemporary experience of health and illness. On the one hand, stillbirth may be considered as a highly individualized experience. On the other hand, societal influences on this event may be observed at both the level of individual meaning and societal structures (Murphy, 2012). My own work with clinical colleagues in this area (Downe et al., 2012, 2013; Kingdon et al., 2015a, 2015b) shows that one of the unintended consequences of the proliferation of reproductive technologies is that reproductive loss is becoming harder to reconcile – at the level of individuals and society.

Stillbirth: a new global controversy?

Despite improvements in general health and developments in maternity care, which include the proliferation of technologies for in utero foetal surveillance during pregnancy and birth, and improvements in some countries, stillbirths nonetheless remain the largest contributor to perinatal mortality rates in many countries. In 2013 there were 142 million recorded births worldwide (Population Reference Bureau, 2013) and for approximately three million of these mother and infant pairs, the baby was recorded as stillborn (WHO, 2014b). In high-resource settings such as the US and the UK, few parents even comprehend that stillbirth is still a problem, but these countries have among the highest stillbirth rates in the developed world (Flenady et al., 2011). In 2011, the leading medical journal *The Lancet* published its first stillbirth series and in so doing drew the world's attention to the unique status of stillbirth, both within medicine and in society (Cousens et al., 2011). A year earlier, the journal *Social Science and Medicine* published a special issue entitled 'Joining-up thinking: loss in childbearing from inter-disciplinary perspectives' that also sought to draw attention to this many-sided problem (physical, medical, psychological, public health, social and economic).

General sociological interest in the relationship between society and mortality has diminished in the Global North in recent years; there are certainly no studies with the scope of Durkheim's examination of suicide from which to draw. Michael Bury and Jonathan Gabe (2004) suggest two reasons for the sociological turn away from mortality. First, there is increasing international awareness that 'the inequalities observed in highly developed countries such as the UK or the US pale into comparison with the health status of populations in developing countries' (Bury and Gabe, 2004: 5). Second, inequalities in health have become more pronounced with respect to morbidity, with a focus on mortality seemingly missing this point. In the case of stillbirth, international estimates do show that more than 75 per cent occur in the developing nations of South Asia and sub-Saharan Africa (WHO, 2014b). But at the same time, in high-income countries around one in every 200 women reaching more than 22 weeks gestation will have a stillborn baby (Flenady et al., 2011). This suggests the need to return to old questions about the ways in which the social has come to be bound up with health outcomes, while simultaneously attending to newer questions about the meaning and experience of stillbirth in societies in which the reproductive technologies promoted by globalized medicine proliferate.

In the case of stillbirth, disparities between socioeconomic, ethnic and age groups reflect wider social inequalities in reproductive and general health, which points to the need to understand the wider structural context. The relationship between poverty, deprivation and mortality was first highlighted as a consequence of rapid industrialization and urbanization across Europe in the nineteenth century, with infant mortality becoming a key indicator of the present and future health of a nation during the twentieth century (Earle et al., 2008). While there have been improvements in the overall rate of stillbirth in many high-income countries over the past 20 years, marked inequalities remain. For example, mothers living in the most deprived areas of the UK are twice as likely to experience stillbirth compared to women living in the least deprived areas (Earle et al., 2008). Globally, the likelihood of stillbirth increases with lower socioeconomic status, even after adjusting for factors such as attendance at antenatal appointments or previous reproductive history, with no evidence of this deprivation gap diminishing (Seaton et al., 2012). Younger women and women from ethnic minorities are also more likely to experience stillbirth, while the social patterning of stillbirth risk among migrant women appears to be variable. Gissler and colleagues' (2009) review of 'Stillbirths and infant deaths among migrants in industrialized countries' shows higher stillbirth rates in some migrant groups but not others. It suggests that mortality risk among babies born to migrants are greatest among refugees, non-European migrants to Europe, and 'foreign-born blacks' to the US, but recommends further work in this area.

Although birth counts (live and dead) circulate as objective 'facts', they are only fixed by the knowledge claims that produce them. The productivity of counting is particularly evident for stillbirth, which is an ambiguous entity, both because of the social norms and stigma that surround it and in relation to other material categories of reproductive loss (particularly miscarriage, but also termination of pregnancy and infanticide). Although the term 'stillbirth' universally indicates a baby born dead, the concept of stillbirth is of Western colloquial origin, where it has multiple definitions across time and place (Haws et al., 2010). In the UK, a stillbirth is currently defined as being 'a baby which has issued forth from its mother after the 24th week of pregnancy and which did not breathe or show any other signs of life' (Still-Birth Act, 1992: Section 41). The gestation of 24 weeks was set as a result of twentieth-century developments in neonatal medicine that improved survival rates of premature babies (prior to 1992 the gestational limit imposed was 28 weeks). Losses before the legal classification of stillbirth are considered miscarriages. In

Australia, stillbirth is defined as the death of a baby after 20 weeks in utero until immediately before birth (Li et al., 2011). However, the WHO does not recognize a stillbirth until 28 weeks gestation (Cousens et al., 2011). This points to the ways in which social classifications produce stillbirth (or not) as the case may be.

Breaking the silence: between individuals, society and medicine

It is widely recognized that stillbirths are underreported, especially in the Global South. In 2014, UNICEF and the WHO launched their *Every Newborn* initiative, which aims to record all stillbirths worldwide as an aid to identification and reduction (UNICEF and WHO, 2014). In the WHO's *Neonatal and Perinatal Mortality* report published in 2007, it was suggested that one of the reasons for underreporting of stillbirths in developing countries is that they are simply not perceived as a problem. However, social science research has found stillbirth is a very real problem for those affected in such countries (Haws et al., 2010; Hough, 2010; van der Sijpt and Notermans, 2010). One illustrative example is the anthropologist Rachel Haws and colleagues' (2010) study in Tanzania, which found that stillbirth is largely hidden because it heightens women's vulnerability to social (stigma, sorcery, marriage breakdown) and physical harm. It is the norm for pregnancies and childbearing losses to be concealed, with women experiencing stillbirth advised not to mourn or grieve, with burial rights and purification practices only evoked if the baby is considered mature.

As illustrated in Figure 2.1, in this particular community of individuals in Tanzania, assessments of maturity are not based on Western biomedical categories of pregnancy loss (i.e., miscarriage, stillbirth and neonatal death), pregnancy gestation or whether or not a baby showed any signs of life at birth, but the visual appearance of the baby in the period after birth. Thus, a stillborn baby that is fully formed, large in size and showing little sign of maceration (deterioration of the foetal skin after death in utero) may be claimed as a mature baby that died after birth (neonatal death), so a mother may outwardly mourn and publicly bury her child (Haws et al., 2010).

The incommensurability between biomedical and local categories of reproductive loss has important implications for efforts to formally identify, record and reduce stillbirth – such as the UNICEF/WHO's *Every Newborn* initiative. Haws and colleagues (2010) suggest these women's concern with their baby's size and skin condition may be sufficient to be able to differentiate between fresh stillbirths (most likely intrapartum deaths) and intrauterine deaths (>12 hours before birth) during verbal autopsies. This is crucial to know when targeting future interventions for prevention and points to the importance of stillbirth as a social and a cultural category as well as a medical one.

The complex social and cultural meanings of stillbirth are equally evident in a North American context. For example, the anthropologist Linda Layne's (2003: 16) *Motherhood Lost* shows how the individual experience of pregnancy loss

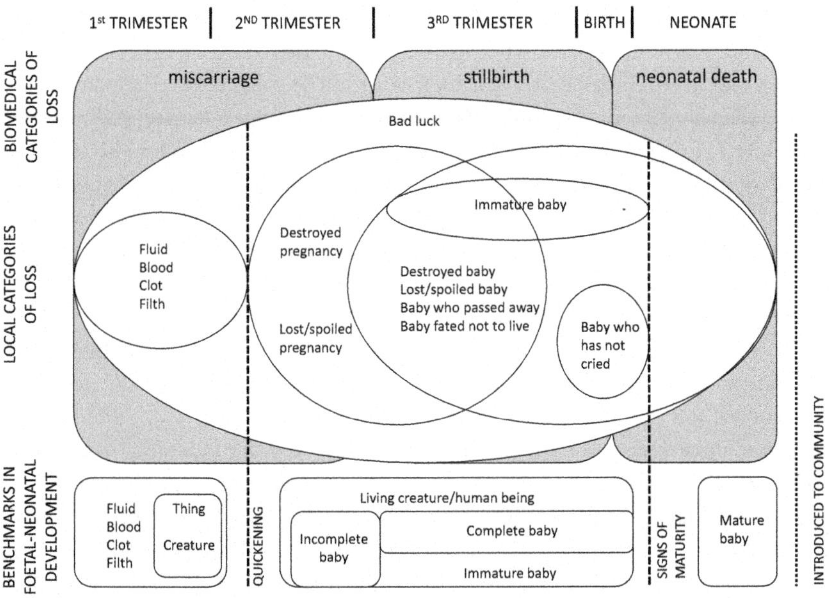

FIGURE 2.1 Biomedical and local categories of pregnancy loss (adapted from Haws et al., 2010).

for middle-class women in the US since the 1980s has been transformed by social change that 'explains in part the rapid growth of the pregnancy loss support movement'. The key change Layne identifies is the increasingly important role of the foetus – the result of changes in abortion legislation, developments in medicine, science and technology, and shifts in family size and the division of labour since the 1970s.[6] Layne suggests that with fewer babies conceived and more pregnancies discontinued by choice, knowledge between women about spontaneous pregnancy loss has diminished. At the same time, changes in the medical management of reproduction have contributed to the emergence of the foetus as a 'patient' from increasingly early gestations. The growing use of commercially available reproductive technologies such as home pregnancy tests and ultrasound imagery are also identified as playing a role in elevating the status of the foetus before birth, which is when personhood was traditionally ascribed.

Precisely because of such developments in reproductive medicine, reproductive success is increasingly seen as something over which individuals have choice and control, despite the aforementioned social differences in stillbirth rates. Deborah Lupton (2012) highlights that pregnancy has become an event surrounded by greater knowledge, expectations of decision-making and awareness of risk as a result of the confluence of forces that Ulrich Beck (1992) has characterized as the 'risk society' (namely, developments in medicine, science and technology and the practices of neoliberal politics). This has the unintended consequence of further stigmatizing women for whom the control of their pregnancy outcome is unattainable.

In a UK context, the sociologist Samantha Murphy (2012) reports that the ten couples and 12 mothers who participated in her study did not expect the pregnancy to end in stillbirth because of: their trust in the capabilities of medicine; the multiple silences surrounding stillbirth; their sense of bodily integrity; and maternal competency. Her argument is that the gendered discourses surrounding parenthood, particularly motherhood, are integral to the framing of the experience of stillbirth, with the unintended consequence of marking men's and women's experiences differently. In detailing mothers' and fathers' lived accounts, Murphy (2012) draws attention to the ideology of the 'moral pregnant mother' 'who is self-sacrificing, nurturing and compliant with medical advice' (Oaks cited in Murphy, 2012: 477). Women who do not live up to this societal ideal run the risk of stigma. Thus, when a pregnancy ends in stillbirth, a woman risks both the loss of identity associated with motherhood, and the loss of the identity of 'moral mother' too.

During interviews, women performed identity work to distance themselves from antenatal behaviours viewed negatively in society (i.e., smoking, drinking, drug-taking, non-compliance with medical advice or non-attendance for antenatal care) and seen as stigmatizing. Men did not. This leads Murphy (2012) to suggest that these women were experiencing what Goffman (1963) referred to as 'felt stigma': internalizing society's dictates and judging themselves by them. As Lupton concludes:

> it is incumbent for critics in public health forums to continue to identify the inequities evident in contemporary medical, public health and popular discourses on pregnant and foetal embodiment and to allow space for consideration of alternatives to placing full responsibility for foetal health and development upon women.
>
> (Lupton, 2012: 338)

Murphy (2012) suggests that this gap in medical knowledge, which means women feel that others blame them for the loss of the baby, necessitates the performance of identity work as 'moral mothers' to counter such stigma. Such performances are only made necessary because of medical knowledge claims about the causes of stillbirth (those that are known) and the dominant societal discourse of neoliberal choice and responsibility for health, which now encompasses pregnancy surveillance and restraint. This points to the complex and contradictory associations between individuals, society, technology and medicine in-the-making of the everyday reality of stillbirth.

Society: a return to the concept's promise

To return to Wright Mills' point that the traditional subject matter of sociology was the total society, what was distinctly sociological about such projects was the continual effort to relate a particular feature of a total society to the whole. Yet he too recognized that 'what was once a promise in these disciplines has become at least a faltering practice' (Wright Mills, 1959: 137). Half a century later, efforts to theorize the social changes of the late twentieth century were to lead others to claim that 'the very idea of society, with all of its ornate indefiniteness, is an idea indebted to the idea of the lost world, for which all sociologies, not just Durkheim's, long' (Lemert, 1995: xvi). Latour perhaps makes this point best when he writes of modernity coming in as many versions as there are thinkers, yet all of its definitions in the guise of society point to the passage of time. As we have seen, Latour's alternative is not to *fix* society, in either sense of the word, but to let questions of the social emerge 'when the ties in which one is entangled begin to unravel' (Latour, 2005: 247).

In their response to the post-societal thesis, the sociologists Anthony Elliot and Bryan Turner (2012: 14) contend that 'with the world now globally refashioned in the image of transnational corporations and agencies – new forms of society, sociality and the social are being constantly, if precariously, reconstituted'. This does not make earlier conceptualizations of society redundant; on the contrary, they are the foundations from which newer questions about society may be built. Elliot and Turner (2012: 15) argue that present-day society – as concept and as lived reality – demands (at least) three senses of society: (1) society as structure, or upper-case Society; (2) society as solidarity, or communities of concern, care and consensus; and (3) society as creative process, or the imaginary dimensions of communication and sociality. They also employ the metaphor of elasticity to explain how social relations may be stretched over place and time, from traditional societies where the thread is thick to internet communities where it becomes thinner and is transitory (with pull of tradition omnipresent). In so doing, the society concept is being transformed once more, and in such a way that celebrates its multiplicity and fluidity as key to understanding the world in which we all live and die.

Conclusion

Many of the ideas about society presented in this chapter are the product of particular transformations in the Western world. This chapter is not advocating that we take what has gone before uncritically as we weave the next generation's lattice-work of tensions between the individual and society, but that we build on it. Despite the relative lack of social science research in high-, middle- or low-income countries investigating stillbirth, the available studies do offer detailed sociocultural insights into the social meanings and expectations concerning reproduction that shape the everyday realities that national and international reproductive health policy seek to address. They employ social science concepts that feature as chapters in this book (culture, society, kinship, magic), among others,[7] to explicate how experience and meaning differ for people with unequal access to material and social resources, due to hierarchies in class, gender, ethnicity and place in the global economy. In so doing, they shed light on what is missing from epidemiological and medical studies of stillbirth that can enhance collective understanding and action.

The question of morality lies at the heart of Durkheim's sociology and reminds us 'not only that there are forms of social solidarity that no individual can live without, but emergent forms of individualism are accompanied by new forms of social interdependence' (Gane, 2014: 1104). The challenge for sociologists is to ensure that the new theoretical agendas for the society concept are interwoven into more applied research into health, technology and medicine. There has never been a more fertile opportunity to build on the theoretical and conceptual resources of the social sciences than the present period offers us to make a difference in the quality of human life.

Notes

1 While at the same time noting attempts to dig up these foundations (Latour, 2005), or to get out of the building game entirely (Lyotard, 1984 [1979]).

2 Positivism, its rise and fall, is perhaps the most noteworthy feature of the social sciences over the past 200 years. Its central assumption is that we could apply the principles of the natural sciences to systematically study various aspects of human life, and as a result improve the lot of humankind through the creation of a new rational order. The promise of positivism was both an exciting and radical new idea for nineteenth-century thinkers. Although it has been increasingly questioned since the middle of the twentieth century, it is nevertheless, 'hard to imagine any social or human scientific approach which does not draw from or develop its ideas in opposition to the positivist approach' (Smith, 2003: 75).

3 'A social fact is any way of acting, whether fixed or not, capable of exerting over the individual an external constraint; or: which is general over the whole of a given society whilst having an existence of its own, independent of its individual manifestations' (Durkheim, 1982 [1895]: 59).

4 Around the same time as Parsons developed his approach to structural functionalism and notions of society based on consensus, the Frankfurt School of critical theory, drawing from Karl Marx, was developing conceptions of society as characterized by conflict.

5 Karl Marx's notion of social class and theories of socioeconomic inequalities between classes are one of the key ways in which we have come to understand society (Table 2.12). The absence of any lengthy discussion of Marx in this chapter is not to dismiss this contribution; on the contrary, his writings provide the foundations for Chapter 4.

6 The precedent for the role of the foetus in public imagery was set on 30 April 1965, when Lennart Nilsson's photograph of an 18-week-old (dead) foetus within in its amniotic sac featured on the cover of *Life* magazine.

7 For example, 'stratified reproduction' (Colen, 1986).

References

Beck, U. (1992) *Risk Society: Towards a New Modernity*. London: Sage.

Beck, U. and Beck-Gernsheim, E. (2002) *Individualization: Institutionalized Individualism and its Social and Political Consequences*. London: Sage.

Bourdieu, P. (1977) *Outline of a Theory of Practice*. Translated by R. Nice. Cambridge, MA: Cambridge University Press.

Brassolotto, J., Raphael, D. and Baldeo, N. (2014) Epistemological barriers to addressing the social determinants of health among public health professionals in Ontario, Canada: a qualitative inquiry. *Critical Public Health*, 24(3): 321–336.

Bury, M. and Gabe, M. (2004) *The Sociology of Health and Illness*. London: Routledge.

Campbell, T. (1981) *Seven Theories of Human Society*. Oxford: Clarendon Press.

Colen, S. (1986) 'Like a mother to them': stratified reproduction and West Indian childcare workers and employers in New York. In F.D. Ginsberg and R. Rapp (eds.), *Conceiving the New World Order: the Global Politics of Reproduction*. Berkeley, CA: University of California Press, 78–102.

Commission on Social Determinants of Health (2008) *Closing the Gap in a Generation: Health Equity Through Action on the Social Determinants of Health*, Final Report of the Commission on Social Determinants of Health. Geneva: World Health Organization.

Comte, A. and Martineau, H. (2009 [1853]) *The Positive Philosophy of Auguste Comte*, Vol. 2. New York: Cambridge University Press.

Cousens, S., Blencowe, H., Stanton, C., Chou, D., Ahmed, S., Steinhardt, L., Creanga, A.A., Tunçalp, Ö., Balsara, Z.P., Gupta, S., Say, L. and Lawn, J.E. (2011) National, regional, and worldwide estimates of stillbirth rates in 2009 with trends since 1995: a systematic analysis. *The Lancet*, 377: 1319–1330.

Dahlgren, G. and Whitehead, M. (1992) *Policies and Strategies to Promote Equity in Health*. Copenhagen: World Health Organization, Regional Office for Europe.

Downe, S., Kingdon, C., Kennedy, R., Norwell, H., McLaughlin, M. and Heazell, A. (2012) Post-mortem examination after stillbirth: views of UK-based practitioners. *European Journal of Obstetrics and Gynecology*, 162(1): 33–37.

Downe, S., Schmidt, E., Kingdon, C. and Heazell, A.E.P. (2013) Bereaved parents' experiences of stillbirth in UK hospitals: qualitative interview study. *BMJ Open*, 3(2).

Durkheim, É. (1952 [1897]) *Suicide: a Study in Sociology*. Translated by J.A. Spaulding and G. Simpson. London: Routledge and Kegan Paul Ltd.

Durkheim, É. (1960 [1893]) *The Division of Labor in Society*. Translated by G. Simpson. Illinois: The Free Press of Glencoe.

Durkheim, É. (1982 [1895]) *The Rules of the Sociological Method*. Basingstoke: Macmillan.

Earle, S., Foley, P., Komaromy, C. and Lloyd, C.E. (2008). Conceptualizing reproductive loss: a social sciences perspective. *Human Fertility*, 11(4): 259–262.

Elliot, A. and Turner, B.S. (2012) *On Society*. Cambridge: Polity Press.

Flenady, V., Middleton, P., Smith, G.C., Duke, W., Japp Erwich, J., Khong, T.Y., Neilson, J., Ezzati, M., Koopmans, L., Ellwood, D., Fretts, R. and Frøen, J.F. (2011) Stillbirths: the way forward in high-income countries. *The Lancet*, 377: 1703–1717.

Frisby, D. and Sayer, D. (1986) *Society*. London: Tavistock.

Gane, N. (2014) Sociology and neoliberalism: a missing history. *Sociology*, 48(6): 1092–1106.

Giddens, A. (1971) *Capitalism and Modern Social Theory*. Cambridge: Cambridge University Press.

Giddens, A. (1984) *The Constitution of Society*. Cambridge: Polity.

Giddens, A. (1990) *The Consequences of Modernity*. Stanford, CA: Stanford University Press.

Gissler, M., Alexander, S., Macfarlane, A., Small, R., Stray-Pedersen, B., Zeitlin, J., Zimbeck, M. and Gagnon, A. (2009) Stillbirths and infant deaths among migrants in industrialized countries. *Acta Obstetricia et Gynecologica Scandinavica*, 88: 134–148.

Goffman, E. (1959) *The Presentation of Self in Everyday Life*. London: Penguin.

Goffman, E. (1963) *Stigma: Notes on the Management of Spoiled Identity*. Prentice-Hall.

Green, J. (2010) The WHO Commission on Social Determinants of Health. *Critical Public Health*, 20(1): 1–4.

Haws, R.A., Mashasi, I., Mrisho, M., Schellenberg, J.A., Darmstadt, G.L. and Winch, P.J. (2010) These are not good things for other people to know: how rural Tanzanian women's experiences of pregnancy loss and early neonatal death may impact survey data quality. *Social Science and Medicine*, 71(10): 1764–1772.

Hough, C.A. (2010) Loss in childbearing among Gambia's kanyalengs: using a stratified reproduction framework to expand the scope of sexual and reproductive health. *Social Science and Medicine*, 71(10): 1757–1763.

Hughes, J.A., Sharrock, W.W. and Martin, P.J. (2003) *Understanding Classical Sociology: Marx, Weber, Durkheim*. London: Sage.

Kingdon, C., Givens, J., O'Donnell, E. and Turner, M. (2015a) Seeing and holding baby: systematic review of clinical management and parental outcomes following stillbirth. *BIRTH: Issues in Perinatal Medicine*. Article first published online 25 June 2015.

Kingdon, C., O'Donnell E., Givens, J. and Turner, M. (2015b) The role of healthcare professionals in encouraging parents to see and hold their stillborn baby: a meta-synthesis of qualitative studies. *PLoS ONE*, 10(7).

Krieger, N. (1994) Epidemiology and the web of causation: has anyone seen the spider? *Social Science and Medicine*, 39(7): 887–903.

Latour, B. (2005) *Reassembling the Social: An Introduction to Actor-Network-Theory*. Oxford: Oxford University Press.

Layne, L. (2003) *Motherhood Lost: A Feminist Account of Pregnancy Loss in America*. New York: Routledge.

Lee, D. and Newby, H. (1989) *The Problem of Sociology*. London: Unwin Hymen.

Lemert, C. (1995) *Sociology after the Crisis*. Boulder, CA: Westview.

Li, Z., McNally, L., Hilder, L. and Sulivan, E. (2011) *Australia's Mothers and Babies 2009*, Perinatal Statistics Series No. 25 Cat. No. PER 52. Sydney: AIHW National Perinatal Epidemiology and Statistics Unit.

Luhmann, N. (1997) Globalization or world society: how to conceive of modern society. *International Review of Sociology*, 7(1): 67–80.

Lupton, D. (2012) 'Precious cargo': foetal subjects, risk and reproductive citizenship. *Critical Public Health*, 22(3): 329–340.

Lyotard, J.F. (1984 [1979]) *The Postmodern Condition: A Report on Knowledge*. Translated by G. Bennington and B. Massumi. Manchester: Manchester University Press.

Marmot, M. and Wilkinson, R. (2006) *Social Determinants of Health*, 2nd edn. Oxford: Oxford University Press.

Marx, K. (1988 [1848]) *The Communist Manifesto*. New York: Norton.

Morrison, K. (2006) *Marx, Durkheim, Weber: Formations of Modern Social Thought*, 2nd edn. London: Sage.

Murphy, S. (2012). Reclaiming a moral identity: stillbirth, stigma and 'moral mothers'. *Midwifery*, 28(4): 476–480.

Nisbet, R. (1993) Society. In W. Outhwaite (ed.), *The Blackwell Companion of Modern Social Thought*. Oxford: Blackwell, 640–642.

Outhwaite, W. (2006) *The Future of Society*. Oxford: Blackwell.

Parsons, T. (1937) *The Structure of Social Action*, Vols. 1 and 2. New York: The Free Press.

Parsons, T. (1951) *The Social System*. London: Routledge and Kegan Paul Ltd.

Parsons, T. (1966) *Societies: Evolutionary and Comparative Perspectives*. New Jersey: Prentice Hall.

Population Reference Bureau (2013) World Population Data Sheet. Available at: www.prb.org/pdf13/2013-population-data-sheet_eng.pdf.

Preda, A. and Voigt, K. (2015) The social determinants of health: why should we care? *American Journal of Bioethics*, 15(3): 25–36.

Raphael, D. (2011) A discourse analysis of the social determinants of health. *Critical Public Health*, 21(2): 221–236.

Schofield, T. (2007) Health inequity and its social determinants: a sociological commentary. *Health Sociology Review*, 16(2): 105–114.

Seaton, S.E., Field, D.J., Draper, E.S., Manktelow, B.N., Smith, G.C.S., Springett, A. and Smith, L.K. (2012) Socioeconomic inequalities in the rate of stillbirths by cause: a population-based study. *BMJ Open*, 2012(2).

Simmel, G. (1992 [1895]) Sociology lectures, in D. Frisby, *Simmel and Since*. London: Routledge.

Smith, M. (2003) *Social Science in Question*. London: Sage.

Spencer, H. (1897 [1876]) *The Principles of Sociology*, 3rd edn. London: Williams and Norgate.

Still-Birth (Definition) Act (1992). London: HMSO.

Tarde, G. (2008 [1899]) *Social Laws: An Outline of Sociology*. Translated by H.C. Warren. Whitefish, MT: Kessinger Publishing.

Tönnies, F. (1963 [1887]) *Community and Society (Gemeinschaft und Gesellschaft)*. Translated and edited by C.P. Loomis. New York: Harper & Row.

Townsend, P. and Davidson, N. (1992 [1980]) *Inequalities in Health: The Black Report and the Health Divide*. London: Penguin.

UNICEF and WHO (2014). *Every Newborn: An Action Plan to End Preventable Deaths*. Available at: www.everynewborn.org/every-newborn-action-plan.

Urry, J. (2000) *Sociology Beyond Societies*. London, Routledge.

van der Sijpt, E. and Notermans, C. (2010) On social sorrows and strategies surrounding pregnancy loss in Cameroon. *Medical Anthropology Quarterly*, 24(3): 381–398.

Wallerstein, I. (1986) Societal development, or development of the world system? In M. Albrow and E. King (eds.), *Globalization, Knowledge and Society*, London: Sage, 157–171.

Weber, M. (1978) *Economy and Society*. Berkeley, CA: University of California Press.

Whitehead, M. (1992 [1987]) *The Health Divide*. Harmondsworth: Penguin.

WHO (2007) *Neonatal and Perinatal Mortality: Country, Regional and Global Estimates*. Geneva: World Health Organization.

WHO (2014a) *Review of Social Determinants of Health and the Health Divide in the WHO European Region*. Copenhagen: World Health Organization.

WHO (2014b) Stillbirths. Available at: www.who.int/reproductivehealth/topics/maternal_perinatal/stillbirth/en.

Wright Mills, C. (1959) *The Sociological Imagination*. Oxford: Oxford University Press.

3

MAGIC

Kirsten Bell

> Nowhere is the duality of natural and supernatural causes divided by a line so thin and intricate, yet, if carefully followed up, so well-marked, decisive, and instructive, as in the two most fateful forces of human destiny: health and death.
>
> Bronisław Malinowski, *Magic, Science and Religion*

Introduction

Central to the operation of contemporary biomedicine is one basic assumption: that certain actions – the administration of particular drugs, a surgical intervention and so on – will produce certain effects. These effects, it is supposed, are immutable: fixed across time and space. In the worldview of biomedicine there is little room for *meaning*. Biomedicine works whether you believe it does or not. No acts of propitiation are required; no charms, rituals or incantations are necessary. Although the status of science has ensured that biomedicine has become the standard against which other medical systems are measured, such systems generally exhibit different kinds of specificity in their reasoning about cause and effect (Csordas, 1989). While many of us adhere to the conviction that our system of knowledge reflects the natural order (Good, 1994), the lines we have drawn between 'natural' and 'supernatural' causes are not universally recognized; nor is much stock placed on our insistence on drawing clear boundaries between signs and things.

These aetiological differences in understandings of health and illness were of immense interest to social scientists long before medical anthropology and sociology emerged as distinct subfields. Anthropology, in particular, has always been centrally concerned with how human beings understand and explain the world around them, a preoccupation that can be traced to the discipline's roots in Enlightenment philosophy, with its concern with rationality and reason (Kapferer, 2002; Tambiah, 1990; see also Chapter 1 for further discussion). Indeed, Bruce Kapferer (2002) argues that anthropology initially established itself as the 'science of unreason', primarily because this quality was understood to constitute the defining characteristic of the discipline's core subject matter: the Other.[1]

The 'primitives' of the nineteenth-century European imagination were irrational, illogical and obsessed with occult forces, in perceived contrast to Europeans themselves, who were deemed to be ruled by science. Thus, debates raged about the relationship between magic, religion and science – topics that were seen to illuminate, in turn, the larger relationship between 'primitive' and 'civilized' society. Although the postmodern, postcolonial turn has sometimes led to a tendency to dismiss these early works, the questions they raised – questions about the foundations of religion, the underlying features of the human psyche and the very nature of science itself – remain of central import (Kapferer, 2002). By taking readers back through these debates, I hope to explicate their salience for contemporary studies of health, medicine and illness and shed light on how this subject matter might be fruitfully approached.

The initial part of the chapter explores the ways in which early scholars conceptualized the relationship between science, magic and religion, and the insights generated by the efforts of the subsequent generation of anthropologists to 'test' their theories. I then examine the increasingly prominent role that the concept of ritual came to play in studies of magic and religion, although such work continued to exhibit a marked preoccupation with questions of rationality and causality – an orientation challenged by the *efficacy* of ritual in healing. Finally, I consider the implications of these insights for contemporary studies of health and medicine, focusing on conceptions of cancer and its treatment as a means of teasing out the problems with notions of causality embedded in science and medicine.

Explaining the cause–effect relationship

Influenced by Edward Tylor's evolutionary model of culture (see Chapter 1), it was Sir James Frazer (1994 [1890]) who provided the most influential early attempt to differentiate magic, science and religion. Although he asserted a clear distinction between magic and science, Frazer suggested that there were a number of parallels between the two. In his words:

> The analogy between the magical and scientific conceptions of the world is close. In both of them the succession of events is assumed to be perfectly regular and certain, being determined by immutable laws, the operation of which can be foreseen and calculated precisely; the elements of caprice, of chance and of accident are banished from the course of nature.
>
> (Frazer, 1994 [1890]: 45)

However, according to Frazer, the 'primitives' who wielded magic misconceived the particular laws that governed nature through a series of mistaken associations. Magic was therefore the 'bastard sister of science' (1994 [1890]: 46). For Frazer, religion differed from both magic and science in that it involved a belief in higher powers and an attempt to propitiate them; it was superior to magic in its awareness of humankind's impotence in certain matters, although he believed it would ultimately fade to irrelevance in the face of science.

Unconvinced by Frazer's framework,[2] Émile Durkheim (1969 [1915]) posited a rather different typology, one in which religion and magic were aligned along the same axis *in opposition to* science. In Durkheim's view, both religion and magic were characterized by beliefs and rituals oriented towards the sacred and served to maintain social cohesion and integration. Science, on the other hand, was preoccupied with the profane.[3] This allowed him to disclaim any real conflict between religion and science, because he saw them as oriented to entirely different phenomena. However, although Durkheim argued that magic was 'hardly distinguishable' from religion (1969 [1915]: 58), he nevertheless suggested several lines of demarcation. First, magic was distinguished by the technical and utilitarian ends to which it was directed;[4] second, religion was communitarian, whereas magic did not bind together those who practiced it: 'there is no Church of magic' (1969 [1915]: 60). Thus, although Frazer and Durkheim differed in their view of the functions of magic, in their typologies, science was the exclusive provenance of civilized 'man'.

Less interested in the specific relationship between magic and religion, the French philosopher Lucien Lévy-Bruhl (1923) further pursued these questions about the nature of 'civilized' and 'primitive' mentalities. Although later scholars were quick to characterize his arguments as racist,[5] Lévy-Bruhl refused to accede to the dominant view of the period (and championed by Frazer) that 'primitives' were mentally inferior to Europeans and insisted that their forms of thought must be understood on their own terms. Observing the tendency of 'primitives' to attribute the causes of phenomena to mystical powers and their lack of interest in (from our point of view) self-evident causal connections, Lévy-Bruhl argued:

> This lack of curiosity does not arise from intellectual torpor or from mental weakness either. Strictly speaking, it is no lack… it has not a 'deficient' or 'negative' reason; it has an actual and positive one. It is the direct and necessary consequence of the fact that primitives live, think, feel, move and act in a world which, in a great many ways, does not coincide with ours.
>
> (Lévy-Bruhl, 1923: 59)

Contra Durkheim, Lévy-Bruhl posited that the leap from what we would call 'natural' to 'supernatural' causes occurred because these realms were not differentiated. In his words, 'The primitive makes no distinction between this world and the other, between what is actually present to sense, and what is beyond' (1923: 32). Thus, what we would call a 'cause' was understood more along the lines of an 'opportunity' – an instrument that served occult powers. For Lévy-Bruhl, this difference in thought-style became most evident in the realm of phenomena that Europeans characterized as 'accidental' or 'coincidental', which were always understood as the manifestation of a mystic power.

Beyond 'armchair' theories

The typologies promulgated by Frazer, Durkheim and Lévy-Bruhl were put to the test by the subsequent generation of anthropologists working in societies where conceptions of magic, witchcraft and sorcery were commonplace. However, those who moved beyond the armchair soon troubled these distinctions drawn between the natural and supernatural, the sacred and profane, cause and effect, and primitive and civilized. Although a number of anthropologists conducted relevant studies, I want to focus here on the work of three particularly influential figures: Bronisław Malinowski, E.E. Evans-Pritchard and Claude Lévi-Strauss.

Malinowski's (1948 [1925]) view of magic shared features in common with both Frazer and Durkheim, although he was strongly motivated by a desire to wrestle the concept of magic from the evolutionism that underwrote prevailing theories – a larger agenda he shared with his American colleague Franz Boas (see Chapter 1). In *Magic, Science and Religion*, Malinowski's key interest was in challenging the assumption that so-called 'primitive man' was unreasoning, devoid of the power to abstract, and with no clear conception of substance and attribute, or cause and effect (Malinowski, 1948 [1925]: 25). Drawing on his fieldwork in the Trobriand Islands, Malinowski observed that ritual and practical work in the realm of farming and fishing generally went hand-in-hand, but this did not mean that Islanders *confused* magic and science. In his words:

> He [the Trobriand Islander] knows as well as you do that there are natural conditions and causes, and by his observations he knows also that he is able to control these natural forces by mental and physical effort... His experience has taught him also, on the other hand, that in spite of all his forethought and beyond all his efforts there are agencies and forces which one year bestow unwanted and unearned benefits of fertility, making everything run smooth and well... and another year again the same agencies bring ill luck and bad chance, pursue him from beginning till end and thwart his most strenuous desires and best-founded knowledge. To control these influences and these only he employs magic.
>
> (Malinowski, 1948 [1925]: 28–29)

Malinowski argued that Trobriand Islanders made a clear-cut distinction between well-known and natural sets of conditions and the domain of unaccountable and adverse influences – the former were dealt with via scientific knowledge and the latter by magic. For Malinowski, magic was a functional response to uncertainty

(Parsons, 1954: 203); thus, magical rituals were limited to contexts where rational techniques could not be relied upon to produce a certain outcome.

However, although Malinowski posited a conceptual distinction between the natural and the supernatural, rational techniques and ritual, and science and magic, his account made it clear that these phenomena bled into each other, a situation especially evident in the realms of health and sickness. According to Malinowski, although Islanders knew that natural forces could negatively affect the body and that old age led to bodily decay, most cases of illness and death were ascribed to sorcery. In particular, the more closely the case in question related to the person experiencing it, the less likely it would be considered natural. Malinowski (1948 [1925]: 32) explained this apparent discrepancy as follows: 'To the most rational of civilized men health, disease, the threat of death, float in a hazy emotional mist, which seems to become denser and more impenetrable as the fateful forms approach.' However, it also suggested that the lines between science and magic, and the natural and the supernatural, were fuzzier than his account implied.

This intrinsic fuzziness became even more apparent in Evans-Pritchard's (1976 [1937]) work on witchcraft and magic among the Azande. On the face of it, Evans-Pritchard's analysis shared much in common with Malinowski's insofar as he emphasized the role of witchcraft in dealing with unfortunate, chance events. To reproduce an oft-quoted passage:

> If blight seizes the ground-nut crop it is witchcraft; if the bush is vainly scoured for game it is witchcraft; if women laboriously bale water out of a pool and are rewarded by but a few small fish it is witchcraft; if termites do not rise when their swarming is due and a cold useless night is spent in waiting for their flight it is witchcraft… if, in fact, any failure or misfortune falls upon anyone at any time and in relation to any of the manifold activities of his life it may be due to witchcraft.
>
> (Evans-Pritchard, 1976 [1937]: 18)

However, where Evans-Pritchard's analysis veered sharply from Malinowski's was that in the latter's account, magic and science were compartmentalized, with magic 'kicking in' when rational techniques couldn't fully account for phenomena. In Evans-Pritchard's analysis, no clear separation was possible and he suggested that Zande notions of witchcraft were fundamentally 'incompatible' with European modes of thought (Evans-Pritchard, 1976 [1937]: 31).

As Jack Goody (1961) later noted, although Evans-Pritchard accepted for heuristic purposes the distinction between ritual and empirical action and mystical and 'common-sense' causality, he simultaneously emphasized the difficulties raised by this acceptance. Thus, Evans-Pritchard denied that the Azande distinguished between the 'natural' and 'supernatural' in the European sense. Instead, in his account, 'natural and supernatural forces as we conceive them are inextricably entwined' (Goody, 1961: 151). According to Kapferer (2002), noteworthy in Evans-Pritchard's account was his refusal to reduce magical practice to terms external to it.[6] In this respect, his argument drew explicit inspiration from Lévy-Bruhl's earlier work, although Evans-Pritchard rejected what he took to be the underlying racism of Lévy-Bruhl's account. In Evans-Pritchard's analysis, magic was not treated as a bastardized parallel to science (as in Frazer's rendering) or an adjunct to it (as in Malinowski's account), but as its own system of thought – one that must be understood on its own terms. In Kapferer's (2002: 6) words: 'Evans-Pritchard effectively questioned the intellectualist implication that science (and associated logical rationalism) and magical practice necessarily can be aligned along the same axis.'

Unfortunately, for the most part, subsequent anthropologists interested in magic, science and religion tended to ignore this basic insight. For example, Claude Lévi-Strauss continued to ask ambitious questions about the nature of European and 'savage' thought. However, although critical of the characterization of magic as a 'timid and stuttering form of science' (Lévi-Strauss, 1966: 13), he argued that magic and science were parallel modes of acquiring knowledge, requiring the same sort of mental operations. They differed not in kind but rather in the types of phenomena to which they were directed.

Clearly influenced by Frazer, Durkheim and Lévy-Bruhl, Lévi-Strauss (1966) argued that magical and mythical thought were characterized by a 'science of the concrete'. Thoroughly empirical, this type of thought was based on a series of associations between sensible properties and intangible qualities; for example, a seed in the form of a tooth might be regarded as a safeguard against snakebites ('sympathetic magic' in Frazer's lexicon). For Lévi-Strauss, the practitioner of magic was a 'bricoleur', 'adept at performing a large number of diverse tasks; but unlike the engineer... his universe of instruments is closed and the rules of his game are always to make do with "whatever is at hand"' (1966: 17).

The rise of ritual

Although anthropologists like Lévi-Strauss were interested in the nature of scientific and magical thought, for the most part, questions of science were quite explicitly partitioned off from anthropological studies of magic and religion. One might be forgiven for thinking this segregation would move studies of magic and religion *away* from questions of scientific rationalism, but they remained integral to the ways ritual came to be defined, especially among those of a structural functionalist bent. For A.R. Radcliffe-Brown, ritual acts 'differ from technical acts in having in all instances some expressive or symbolic element in them' (in Goody, 1961: 152). In other words, ritual was, by definition, an action where the nature of the means–end relationship was symbolic rather than intrinsic (Goody, 1961).

However, as Goody (1961) pointed out, such criteria for segregating ritual phenomena were derived not from the actor's point of view, but from the *observer's* assessment of what was intrinsic.[7] In his words,

> The attribution of a 'symbolic' or 'expressive' element to ritual or religious (i.e. 'non-rational') behaviour often turned out to be no more than a way of announcing that the observer is unable to make sense of an action in terms of an intrinsic means-end relationship, a 'rational' cause and effect nexus, and has therefore to assume that the action in question stands for something other than it appears to; in other words, that it expresses or is symbolic of something else.
>
> (Goody, 1961: 156)

It is this sense of patterned action that fails to accomplish an observable outcome that has become central to the term's broader usage[8] (Goody, 1961, 1977).

Kapferer (2004: 38) notes that such accounts treat ritual as a primarily symbolic and representational phenomenon: a 'technology of traditional, relatively static societies, a mechanism for their reproduction, and as a means for the delusion and mystification of populations, which facilitated the legitimacy of dominant orders'. This view of ritual pervades the work of his fellow colleagues in the Manchester School, including Max Gluckman (1954), J. Clyde Mitchell (1956) and Max Marwick (1965), although their Marxist orientation led to a focus on rituals as a manifestation of social struggle and political conflict. However, it was a member of the Manchester School, Victor Turner, who was chiefly responsible for shifting analytic attention from ritual as representation to ritual as *process*.

Signs versus things and the question of ritual efficacy

Although Victor Turner's early writing was heavily influenced by Gluckman's (1954) work on rituals of rebellion, his notion of the 'social drama'[9] initiated an interest in ritual processes and the fundamentally dynamic character of social relations. Turner (1967, 1969, 1974) later drew inspiration from Arnold Van Gennep (1960 [1908]), who identified a sequence of events typical to most rites of passage: separation, transition (or *limen*) and incorporation. Although Van Gennep endorsed Durkheim's distinction between the sacred and profane, he did not write of ritual in the Durkheimian sense – as a symbolic formation of the social or as an expression of society; instead, he alluded to its ability to facilitate change within society. According to Kapferer (2004: 38), Turner pushed this line of thought well beyond Van Gennep's arguments to recognize 'the capacity of ritual to bring forth and change the very ground of being'. Turner's concentration on the ritual process radically reoriented the anthropological analysis of ritual. Here was an approach that asked heretofore neglected questions about how rituals might be instrumental as well as representational – how they might actually *do* things (Sax, 2010).

These ideas became particularly important for subsequent studies of illness and healing. For example, Kapferer's own work on Sinhalese healing rituals (1983) took up such insights to illuminating effect. Focusing on Sinhalese Buddhists afflicted by demonic attacks, his main concern was with healing rites and their transformational process. While recognizing the social context of demonic disorder (the predominance of female patients, the class bias of demonic exorcism, etc.), Kapferer nevertheless insisted that demonic illness could not be reduced to terms external to it and highlighted the *dynamics* of the exorcisms themselves. In his words,

> Rituals are more than the organized symbolic reflection of central cultural ideas… Rituals act practically upon the world; this is effected through their major defining quality: rituals place ideas in a dominant relation to action and constrain action and experience within them… Rituals can also transform action and experience; this they do by attacking and restructuring the ideas in terms of which action and experience are comprehended. This transformational capacity of ritual is highly evident in healing rites; indeed, their practical efficacy depends on this capacity.
>
> (Kapferer, 1983: 326)

This point is powerfully illustrated in Lévi-Strauss's (1967) essay 'The effectiveness of symbols'. Focusing on a song used by Cuna shamans to ease a difficult childbirth, Lévi-Strauss highlighted the ways in which myth and prosaic reality, the physical and physiological universe, and the external and internal world, became connected through the ritual. He argued that through the song, the intolerable pains of childbirth were rendered acceptable to the birthing mother's mind:

> The sick woman believes in the myth and belongs to a society which believes in it… The sick woman accepts these mythical beings… what she does not accept are the incoherent and arbitrary pains, which are an alien element in her system but which the shaman, calling upon the myth, will integrate within a whole where everything is meaningful. Once the sick woman understands, however, she does more than resign herself; *she gets well.*
>
> (Lévi-Strauss, 1967: 192–193, emphasis added)

Although Lévi-Strauss's account clearly demonstrated the 'thinginess' of signs for the Other (i.e., their ability to affect physiological change in the birthing woman), he rejected the possibility of such entwinement in a Western context – except in the context of psychological ailments – because medicine dealt in things rather than signs. In his words,

> no such thing happens to our sick when the causes of their disease have been explained to them in terms of secretions, germ, or viruses… the relationship

> between germ and disease is external to the mind of the patient, for it is a cause-and-effect relationship; whereas the relationship between monster and disease is internal to his mind.
>
> (Lévi-Strauss, 1967: 193)

Yet, in rejecting what I will call here the 'signiness' of things, Lévi-Strauss's argument was flawed in both specifics and generalities. As Emily Martin (1994) has illustrated, scientific theories about germs and disease are themselves simultaneously cultural models. Moreover, cultural models of how drugs work – and the rituals associated with their administration – have an indisputable effect on how they *actually* work. As William Sax (2010: 7) points out, what makes ritual so interesting is that it negates the modern, scientific episteme. How else can we explain the placebo effect, perhaps the ultimate example of the limitations of the scientific insistence on the separation between signs and things?

Usually translated as 'I shall please', the placebo effect is generally defined as a substance that has an objective effect without containing any specific activity for the condition being treated (Hahn and Kleinman, 1983; Moerman, 1983, 2002).[10] Although the term is often bandied about in a derisive fashion, Ayo Wahlberg (2008) argues that anthropological research by figures such as Evans-Pritchard, Lévi-Strauss and Turner, among others, had an essential role to play in 'decriminalizing' the placebo effect during the course of the twentieth century – i.e., transforming it from the tool of trade of quacks and charlatans into a legitimate and 'real' object of scientific scrutiny. In Wahlberg's (2008: 79) words, 'the concept of the "placebo effect" came to mediate symbolic and somatic concepts of therapeutic efficacy as a kind of spill-over effect measurable "at the end organs"'.

It's because of the placebo effect that drug marketers have to consider the colour of their product and the form in which it is distributed as well as its content. This is because we all 'know' that injections are more powerful than pills, very tiny pills are more powerful than aspirin-style pills, and red pills are stimulants and blue pills are depressants (Moerman, 2002). We know this regardless of the actual content of these medications and, sure enough, presented as 'medicine', a red sugar pill is likely to make us feel more alert and a blue sugar pill will probably have a sedative effect.[11] It is also because of the placebo effect that the 'gold standard' in clinical medicine is the double-blind randomized controlled trial: participants must be as similar as possible and then randomly assigned to the treatment or a placebo; ideally, neither the subjects nor those delivering the treatment should know who received what. How otherwise is the researcher to know that it was the chemical properties of the drug that caused the effect rather than the subject's belief in its efficacy? That such an extraordinary amount of effort has been devoted to containing the placebo effect demonstrates just how important meaning is to medicine, 'in spite of professional (and societal) attempts to expunge meaning and value from the equation of care' (Kleinman, 1988: 30).

Implications for contemporary studies of health and medicine

Byron Good (1994) argues that central to anthropology (although the point holds equally true for sociology) has been a distinction between 'belief' and 'knowledge', with the latter seen to correspond to ideas that accord with objective reality and the former to ideas that have no basis in it. In this formulation, science is the arbiter between the empirically real and the mystical. However, as Good (1994: 27) observes, such 'claims that biomedicine provides straightforward, objective depictions of the natural order, an empirical order of biological universals, external to culture, no longer seem tenable', especially in light of the growing body of scholarship by sociologists, anthropologists and philosophers on the ways scientific knowledge is produced.

Bruno Latour (1993) has called for a *symmetrical* anthropology, arguing that if pre-moderns are said to never distinguish between signs and things (Frazer's and Lévy-Bruhl's argument), *neither do 'We'*. Put more accurately, '"We" do not distinguish between Nature and Society more than "They" make them overlap' (Latour, 1993: 103). Latour points out when the anthropologist comes in from the tropics to study the modern world, 'at first, it thinks it can apply its methods only when Westerners mix up signs and things the way savage thought does' (1993: 100). Confining ourselves to lay perspectives on health and illness, or popular medicine, or complementary and alternative medicine, is one way that anthropologists do this, 'because the question of Nature – that is, of science – is not yet raised' (Latour, 1993: 100). However, Latour's vision of a truly symmetrical anthropology is one where the anthropology of the modern moves from the periphery to the centre: 'their belief system, their technologies, their ethno-sciences' (1993: 100).

If we have learnt anything from the anthropological debates about the nature of magic, ritual and science, it is that we must guard against the following binaries:

Science	Magic/ritual
Rational	Irrational
Things	Signs
Efficacious	Inert
Body	Mind
Nature	Society

However, relinquishing such ideas is no easy task, given the ways such dualisms are embedded in Western thought. As Scheper-Hughes and Lock (1987) note, despite our attempts to study the experience of illness and suffering from an integrated perspective, we find ourselves perpetually trapped by the Cartesian legacy. This is equally true of studies of magic and ritual and other key topics that have captured the attention of social scientists, such as production (see Chapter 4), kinship (see Chapter 5) and the body (see Chapter 7).

Cancer and causality

The extent of the problem can be readily illustrated in studies of a disease where science seems to reach the limits of its knowledge: cancer. Cancer is distinctive insofar as it stems from uncertain causes and its manifestations are multiple (Csordas, 1989). As S. Lochlann Jain observes:

> Too wily to be tethered to a solid noun, the conundrums of cancer match its craftiness. Despite news articles promising a cure… scientists continue to furiously debate how cancer arises, whether it should be studied as one disease or hundreds, whether mice provide adequate research models, and who might benefit from the arsenal of commonplace, if dangerous, cancer treatments such as chemotherapy and radiation.
>
> (Jain, 2013: 2)

In *Malignant: How Cancer Becomes Us*, Jain (2013) demonstrates that cancer is anything *but* an objective thing; instead, it's better understood as a process and social field – one in which the 'facts' of cancer are inseparable from their interpretation. However, efforts to understand lay conceptions of cancer and its treatment have often unwittingly reinscribed these distinctions, as two examples from earlier anthropological research demonstrate.

In her ethnography on the response of a working-class community in Philadelphia to a state-sponsored cancer prevention campaign, Martha Balshem (1993) explores the radical disjuncture between what health promotion workers and the local community 'know' about cancer. The primary goals of community health educators employed on Project CAN-DO were to encourage locals to adopt healthier lifestyle behaviours (stop smoking, improve their diet, undergo regular cancer screening) and to dispel seven 'misconceptions' held about cancer among the local community:

1. There is nothing you can do to prevent cancer.
2. There is cancer hidden in everybody.
3. Cancer can be triggered by a bruise or blow to the body.
4. Cancer is inherited.
5. Surgery can cause cancer to spread.
6. Cancer treatment is worse than the disease itself.
7. Cancer is a death sentence.

For the majority of health educators, these beliefs were evidence of the fatalism and irrationality of the community. However, Balshem focuses on the community resistance to dominant models of cancer control such views entail, where individuals are exhorted to take responsibility for cancer through individual action. She also takes pains to explain that these 'myths' are actually entirely logical and rational interpretations of the available evidence. For example, she observes that there is nothing an individual can do to absolutely guarantee that they won't get cancer, some cancers do in fact develop through a series of precancerous events, and physical trauma may sometimes enhance the growth or spread of pre-existing cancers, etc.

The problem, of course, is that explaining beliefs in this way reduces them to terms external to them. Balshem seems to recognize this herself to some degree, acknowledging in the book's introduction that:

> To date, in my written descriptions of community beliefs about cancer, I had felt it necessary to point out that the community critique is based on fact – an epistemological category distinctively different from being fact. In this and other ways, I had allowed the implication that ultimate knowledge is still always held by medical science.
>
> (Balshem, 1993: 9)

In contemporary anthropological research into health and illness, it's often tempting to translate local beliefs into 'rational' terms. Thus, the anthropologist becomes a kind of cultural mediator (and magician), revealing with a flourish (voilà!) that apparently irrational and superstitious beliefs and rituals are actually rational and logical after all. Such efforts can be a powerful antidote to medical authority, but they also lock us into the rational/irrational frame. Moreover, they ultimately reinforce prevailing knowledge structures. In sum, although a growing number of medical anthropologists have chosen to take medical knowledge and practice itself as the object of anthropological inquiry, many continue to define themselves in the highly circumscribed role of 'cultural broker' (Scheper-Hughes, 1990; Baer et al., 2003). While this role is often necessary and praiseworthy, 'what is not being called into question is the inevitability (nor the technological superiority) of the whole biomedical health enterprise itself' (Scheper-Hughes, 1990: 191).

I should emphasize that the tendency I have identified in Balshem's work is one that I have been equally guilty of myself (and far less reflexive about than Balshem). For example, during an eight-month period of fieldwork conducted at a cancer support group for people with colorectal cancer, I noticed that participants in the group talked about chemotherapy in ways that contradicted its biomedical operation (see Bell, 2009). In particular, they seemed to equate suffering during chemotherapy with efficacy – in other words, the more side-effects they experienced, the better they presumed the treatment was working. They also believed that they had to get the 'full' dose in order for chemotherapy to be effective, and experienced considerable distress when low white blood cell counts meant their treatment was delayed. Intravenous chemotherapy was also understood to be far stronger than oral chemotherapy, and so people often characterized the seriousness of their cancer in relation to the type of treatment they received.

However, from a biomedical perspective, toxicity does not equal gain; instead, chemotherapy is a delicate balancing act *between* toxicity and gain. The goal is to achieve the greatest effect with the least amount of unnecessary harm. But the only means oncologists have to determine this are clinical trials, which produce data on average effects. Thus, the standard chemotherapy regime for patients with stage III colon cancer is much higher than many individual patients need. In consequence, while an insufficient dose or prolonged treatment delays are seen to undermine the effectiveness of therapy, it is standard practice to dose-reduce when patients are exhibiting high-grade toxicities without a perceived compromise in treatment outcomes. Nor is the form of the chemotherapy (oral versus intravenous) associated with the seriousness of the cancer: many forms of oral chemotherapy are just as strong as intravenously delivered drugs.

In light of this disjuncture between a scientific perspective on chemotherapy and that of group members, I argued that these were entirely rational and logical responses to the indeterminacy of chemotherapy. I asserted that people made sense of their experience in terms of other drug models they were familiar with (for example, antibiotics) and in relation to dominant cultural motifs about the efficacy of suffering ('whatever doesn't kill you makes you stronger'). I went on to posit a relatively bounded and internally coherent system of beliefs surrounding chemotherapy. While I don't necessarily disagree with various aspects of my initial analysis, over time I have come to see that I was guilty of precisely the kind of rationalism and cultural brokerage that others have criticized.

As the epigraph from Malinowski suggests, the realms of health and disease are matters of deep existential concern. Where our views diverge is the assumption that the dividing line between natural and supernatural causes (which he acknowledges as 'thin') can be firmly drawn. Simply put, we cannot reduce beliefs about health and illness – whether they involve mystical beings, sympathetic magic, or ideas about the efficacy of suffering – to the problem of reason. There has to be a place in studies of health and medicine for the 'realms of unreason', one that treats such beliefs on their own terms, rather than binding them to the question of rationality. Such beliefs are always contextual and situationally adaptive rather than taking the form of abstract or coherent 'rules'. 'The "system" of ideas and practice of which they are part is constantly immanent, enduringly emergent, differentiating and shifting in response to new circumstances' (Kapferer, 2002: 7).

A related issue with my analysis is that, like Balshem, I was measuring patients' beliefs about chemotherapy *against* biomedical ones – using the biomedical framework as the objective standard, and treating biomedical knowledge as relating exclusively to the realm of 'things' rather than 'signs'. The problem is that biomedical understandings of chemotherapy are simultaneously a cultural model. For example, the notion of a 'side-effect' is itself not a natural way of thinking about the operation of chemotherapy. It is a way of conceptually partitioning the desired actions of drugs (destroying malignant cells) and their undesirable – but equally intrinsic – actions (destroying benign cells). As Nina Etkin (1992: 102) observes in her analysis of the concept of 'side-effects', 'the codification of pharmaco-therapeutic outcomes into "primary action" and "side effect" implies an intuitive and universal logic that simply does not obtain, even in biomedicine'.

If we look beneath the surface of biomedicine to the contexts in which chemotherapy is embedded, we soon see that oncologists themselves do not distinguish between nature and society in quite the mechanical way we might have initially assumed. In other words, our own system is not one based exclusively on the notion of scientifically verifiable cause and effect, although it might at first glance appear to be such. Mary-Jo DelVecchio Good and her colleagues (1990) have highlighted the ways in which American oncological practice is infused with a discourse on 'hope' grounded in an underlying conception about the relationship between the mind and body, and psyche and soma. This oncological discourse on hope structures encounters between physicians and patients, manifested in the importance of instilling and maintaining hope throughout the course of treatment.

DelVecchio Good and her colleagues emphasize that the discourse on hope invoked by physicians is not equivalent to that found in some forms of popular medicine (although it has resonances with it), which emphasize the ways that cancer patients – if they just have enough will power – can heal themselves. Instead, it is more of an agnostic, generalized notion of the value of hope in promoting the patient's recovery. Of equal importance is the *physician's* ability to maintain hope that she can make a difference. This 'political economy of hope' structures not only the individual therapeutic encounter itself, but the larger context of research and funding (see Novas, 2006; Rose, 2007). All this is to suggest that the effects of chemotherapy (and understandings of such) cannot be divorced from the system in which it is embedded and reduced to simplistic notions of cause and effect. Again we see that signs and things refuse to stay in their place, whether the context be lay understandings of chemotherapy *or* biomedical conceptions themselves.

Conclusion

The history of debate about concepts such as magic and science in the social sciences and humanities shows us that it has been difficult to shed Enlightenment concerns about causality, rationality and reason. These concerns are evident in attempts to view magic as a form of bastardized science and the insistence on defining ritual phenomena based on their lack of 'intrinsic' cause–effect relationship. The spectre of science loomed large in these debates, mostly as the implicit standard against which magical phenomena were measured and understood. But those anthropologists who moved beyond the armchair engaged with ethnographic worlds that exceeded their theories and interpretations. These accounts (in some cases implicitly and in other cases explicitly) showed the importance of grappling with phenomena that might otherwise seem 'exotic', 'illogical' or 'irrational', without reducing them to terms external to them. They also challenged notions of causality embedded in science and the separation of signs and things upon which it is founded.

Today, the social sciences continue to grapple with the legacy of this split between belief and knowledge and society and nature, which remains a central conceptual problem in medical anthropology and sociology (Good, 1994). However, the insights generated through earlier studies of magic and ritual are profoundly important for contemporary social scientists wanting to study health and medicine. As Good (1994: 181) observes, such research provides a necessary counter to the dominance of instrumental rationality and the threat it poses to 'human freedom and to our experience of the meaningful, mythological, and transcendent dimensions of illness, healing, and human experience'.

Notes

1 See Stanley Tambiah's (1990) work for a comprehensive examination of the historical, political and philosophical context of anthropological theories of magic, science and religion. As he illustrates, anthropological interest in this topic was strongly influenced by Renaissance philosophy, the Protestant Reformation and Enlightenment concerns, often with very little awareness among anthropologists of the ways in which they imported these concerns into studies of the Other.

2 Durkheim attacked Frazer's work at various points in *The Elementary Forms of Religious Life*, especially the latter's refusal to acknowledge the fundamentally religious nature of totemism and his insistence on characterizing it as a magical system.

3 Durkheim didn't state this directly, but it is implicit in his discussion of science in *The Elementary Forms of the Religious Life*. In this respect, his position differed from that of Frazer and Edward Tylor, who saw religion as a primitive 'survival' that would be eventually relegated to 'the dustbin of history' (Strenski, 2006: 101).

4 Durkheim's definition has some resonance with Frazer's in this respect. Although Durkheim argued that magic was oriented towards sacred beings and beliefs, he suggested that the *questions* it explored were decidedly profane rather than 'speculative'; indeed, for Durkheim ([1915]1969: 58) 'magic takes a sort of professional pleasure in profaning holy things'.

5 Such views are based on a misreading of Lévy-Bruhl's work (see Shore, 1996; Hage, 2012). *Primitive Mentality* is certainly replete with references to 'primitive', 'inferior' and 'prelogical' peoples and Lévy-Bruhl did suggest that the 'primitive mentality' had a limited capacity for innovation and the acquisition of new knowledge. However, in his view, this was because of a style of thought that always assimilated the 'new' into existing experience, rather than any constitutional incapacity – a line of argument not too dissimilar from that later promulgated by Lévi-Strauss (1966). Moreover, unlike the majority of his contemporaries, Lévy-Bruhl was well aware of the problems with the term 'primitive' (see Lévy-Bruhl, 1923: 13).

6 See the work of Byron Good (1994: 11–14) for a contrasting interpretation. Good argues that Evans-Pritchard's work is strongly grounded in the rationality tradition, although he acknowledges that 'Evans-Pritchard's text transcends its empiricist formulation, in particular because of the subtlety of its analysis of Zande reasoning and the location of witchcraft in Zande social relations' (1994: 13). Conversely, de Pina-Cabral (2014: 154) argues: 'Many of the readings of Evans-Pritchard's work on the Azande fail to see that he was attempting to explain how religious thought operates; he was not validating it as being rational or truthful.'

7 Unfortunately, despite the interesting questions he raised in the paper, Goody concluded by attempting to generate his own definition of ritual – one that seemed to contain the very limitations he highlighted insofar as it wedded itself to questions of rationality. However, he later seemed to recant this view, emphasizing the futility of attempts to define ritual and suggesting that the concept itself was so flawed, we would be better off jettisoning it entirely (see Goody, 1977).

8 In common parlance, a 'ritual' is often used to denote a series of formalized but essentially ineffective actions (Sax, 2010).
9 For Turner (1972 [1957]: xvii), a social drama is a social irruption that allows one to 'look beneath the surface of social regularities into the hidden contradictions and conflicts in the system'.
10 Daniel Moerman (2002) suggests that the term 'meaning response' is a more appropriate way of characterizing this phenomenon. As he points out, the problem with the concept of the placebo effect is that it relies on a simplistic, mechanical notion of cause and effect (the very same notion, of course, that has long plagued anthropological definitions of magic and ritual).
11 Unless we happen to be Italian, male and a football fan, or a middle-aged man with erectile problems – see Moerman (2002: 49–50) for an entertaining discussion of the polysemous meanings of blue pills.

References

Baer, H.A., Singer, M. and Susser, I. (2003) *Medical Anthropology and the World System*, 2nd edn. Westport, CT: Praeger Publishers.

Balshem, M. (1993) *Cancer in the Community: Class and Medical Authority*. Washington, DC: Smithsonian Institution.

Bell, K. (2009) 'If it almost kills you that means it's working': cultural models of chemotherapy expressed in a cancer support group. *Social Science and Medicine*, 68(1): 169–176.

Csordas, T.J. (1989) The sore that does not heal: cause and concept in the Navajo experience of cancer. *Journal of Anthropological Research*, 45(4): 457–485.

DelVecchio Good, M-J., Good, B.J., Schaffer, C. and Lind, S.E. (1990) American oncology and the discourse on hope. *Culture, Medicine and Psychiatry*, 14(1): 59–79.

de Pina-Cabral, J. (2014) World: an anthropological examination (part 2). *Hau: Journal of Ethnographic Theory*, 4(3): 149–184.

Durkheim, É. (1969 [1915]) *The Elementary Forms of the Religious Life*. Translated by J.W. Swain. New York: The Free Press.

Etkin, N.L. (1992) 'Side effects': cultural constructions and reinterpretations of western pharmaceuticals. *Medical Anthropology Quarterly*, 6(2): 99–113.

Evans-Pritchard, E.E. (1976 [1937]) *Witchcraft, Oracles, and Magic Among the Azande*. Oxford: Clarendon Press.

Frazer, J. (1994 [1890]) *The Golden Bough: A Study in Magic and Religion*. Oxford: Oxford University Press.

Gluckman, M. (1954) *Rituals of Rebellion in South-East Africa*. Manchester: Manchester University Press.

Good, B.J. (1994) *Medicine, Rationality and Experience: An Anthropological Perspective*. Cambridge: Cambridge University Press.

Goody, J. (1961) Religion and ritual: the definitional problem. *British Journal of Sociology*, 12(2): 142–164.

Goody, J. (1977) Against 'ritual': Loosely structured thoughts on a loosely defined topic. In S.F. Moore and B.G. Myerhoff (eds.), *Secular Ritual*. Assen: Van Gorcum and Comp, 25–35.

Hage, G. (2012) Critical anthropological thought and the radical political imaginary today. *Critique of Anthropology*, 32(3): 285–308.

Hahn, R. and Kleinman, A. (1983) Perspectives of the placebo phenomenon: Belief as pathogen, belief as medicine – 'Voodoo death' and the 'placebo phenomenon' in anthropological perspective. *Medical Anthropology Quarterly*, 14(4): 3–19.

Jain, S.L. (2013) *Malignant: How Cancer Becomes Us.* Berkeley, CA: University of California Press.
Kapferer, B. (1983) *A Celebration of Demons: Exorcism and the Aesthetics of Healing in Sri Lanka.* Oxford: Berg.
Kapferer, B. (2002) Outside all reason: magic, sorcery and epistemology in anthropology. *Social Analysis*, 46(3): 1–30.
Kapferer, B. (2004) Ritual dynamics and virtual practice: beyond representation and meaning. *Social Analysis*, 48(2): 25–54.
Kleinman, A.M. (1988) *The Illness Narratives: Suffering, Healing and the Human Condition.* New York: Basic Books.
Latour, B. (1993) *We Have Never Been Modern.* Translated by C. Porter. Cambridge, MA: Harvard University Press.
Lévi-Strauss, C. (1966) *The Savage Mind.* Translated by G. Weidenfeld. Chicago: University of Chicago Press.
Lévi-Strauss, C. (1967) The effectiveness of symbols. In *Structural Anthropology.* Translated by C. Jacobsen and B.G. Shoepf. New York: Anchor Books, 181–201.
Lévy-Bruhl, L. (1923) *Primitive Mentality.* Translated by L.A. Clare. London: George Allen and Unwin Ltd.
Malinowski, B. (1948 [1925]) *Magic, Science and Religion and Other Essays.* Prospect Heights, IL: Waveland Press.
Martin, E. (1994) *Flexible Bodies: The Role of Immunity in American Culture from the Days of Polio to the Age of AIDS.* Boston, MA: Beacon Press.
Marwick, M. (1965) *Sorcery in its Social Setting: A Study of the Northern Rhodesian Cewâ.* Manchester: Manchester University Press.
Mitchell, J.C. (1956) *The Yao Village: A Study in the Social Structure of a Malawian People.* Manchester: Manchester University Press.
Moerman, D. (1983) Perspectives of the placebo phenomenon: general medical effectiveness and human biology – placebo effects in the treatment of ulcer disease. *Medical Anthropology Quarterly*, 14(4): 3–16.
Moerman, D. (2002) *Meaning, Medicine and the 'Placebco Effect'.* Cambridge: Cambridge University Press.
Novas, C. (2006) The political economy of hope: patients' organizations, science and biovalue. *BioSocieties*, 1(3): 289–305.
Parsons, T. (1954) *Essays in Sociological Theory.* Glencoe, IL: The Free Press.
Rose, N. (2007) *The Politics of Life Itself: Biomedicine, Power, and Subjectivity in the Twenty-First Century.* Princeton, NJ: Princeton University Press.
Sax, W.S. (2010) Ritual and the problem of efficacy. In W.S. Sax, J. Quack, and J. Weinhold (eds.), *The Problem of Ritual Efficacy.* Oxford: Oxford University Press, 3–16.
Scheper-Hughes, N. (1990) Three propositions for a critically applied medical anthropology. *Social Science and Medicine*, 30(2): 189–197.
Scheper-Hughes, N. and Lock, M.M. (1987) The mindful body: a prolegomenon to future work in medical anthropology. *Medical Anthropology Quarterly*, 1(1): 6–41.
Shore, B. (1996) *Culture in Mind: Culture, Cognition, and the Problem of Meaning.* Oxford: Oxford University Press.
Strenski, I. (2006) *Thinking about Religion: A Reader.* Hoboken, NJ: Wiley-Blackwell.
Tambiah, S.J. (1990) *Magic, Science, Religion, and the Scope of Rationality.* Cambridge: Cambridge University Press.
Turner, V.W. (1967) *The Forest of Symbols: Aspects of Ndembu Ritual.* Ithaca: Cornell University Press.
Turner, V.W. (1969) *The Ritual Process: Structure and Anti-Structure.* New York: Aldine de Gruyter.

Turner, V.W. (1972 [1957]) *Schism and Continuity in an African Society: A Study of Ndembu Village Life*. Manchester: University of Manchester Press.

Turner, V.W. (1974) *Dramas, Fields and Metaphors: Symbolic Action in Human Society*. Ithaca: Cornell University Press.

Van Gennep, A. (1960 [1908]) *The Rites of Passage*. Translated by M.B. Vizedom and G.L. Caffee. London: Routledge and Kegan Paul.

Wahlberg, A. (2008) Above and beyond superstition – Western herbal medicine and the decriminalizing of placebo. *History of the Human Sciences*, 21(1): 77–101.

4

PRODUCTION

Carol Kingdon

> The mode of production of material life conditions the general process of social, political, and intellectual life.
>
> Karl Marx, *A Contribution to the Critique of Political Economy*

Introduction

Since the late eighteenth century, and the transition from agricultural-based production to industrial technology-based production in Western Europe, the concept of production has been employed as a means of understanding the character of social relations in different societies. This chapter takes up the concept of production, principally in relation to human reproduction, to explore the shifting boundaries between the hitherto curative practices of medicine, and the present-day trend for enhancement of life, lifestyle and self-identity through medicine. Recent changes in late twentieth and early twenty-first century forms of Westernized neoliberal capitalism have been theorized by some (i.e., Bauman, 2007) more in relation to individual consumption, with less attention paid to the relations between the market and rise of consumerism. Health and healthcare constitute one of the largest, fastest-growing and complex markets in the world, yet neither per capita government health expenditure nor private health provider income guarantee quality of care, improved health outcomes or access to reproductive healthcare in times of need. In 2012 the United States spent 17 per cent of its gross domestic product (total GDP $16.24 trillion) on healthcare, yet is one of only two high-income countries without universal healthcare provision (World Bank, 2014). This chapter is critical of the ever-increasing coalescence between the pursuit of profit *and* the intensification of the relationships between the market, medicine, science and technology.

The first part of the chapter traces the co-constituted conceptual heritages of production and consumption from Karl Marx to the present day, including how they have been taken up in theories on 'medicalization' and 'biomedicalization'. The chapter then turns attention to how feminist scholarship has reconceived production in relation to reproduction. Formulations of reproduction operate both at the level of society (i.e., social norms, values, inequalities) and the reproduction of human life (i.e., fertility, childbirth), with general social science interest in production facilitating a specifically feminist interest in human reproduction. In recent decades, the reproductive body (male and female) has become increasingly commercialized and rendered perfectible through science, medicine, technology, the market and the media, with demand, health and healthcare consequences purportedly a matter of individual choice. Through a case study of childbirth, and planned caesarean birth in particular, the enduring value of the production concept is highlighted wherever capitalism is the key organizing principle of society.

Foundations of an approach to production

For Marx, whose influence endures across the social sciences, production was *the* defining social activity from which all human relations are organized and the processes of social change originate. According to Marx, it is through society (see Chapter 2) that human beings are history-makers through material activity and labour. What is more, the history we as humans make is what we think and work from to orchestrate change. Marx used the term 'mode of production' to refer to the economic base of society, from which, he theorized, all other aspects of society are ultimately, but not exclusively, determined. In *A Contribution to the Critique of Political Economy*, Marx wrote: 'we can designate the Asiatic, ancient, feudal and the modern industrial modes of production as so many epochs in the process of the economic formation of society' (1977 [1859]: 21). Thus, for Marx, industrial capitalism was just one 'mode of production' in his evolutionary schema of social structures and social change. For Marx, the capitalist mode of production is comprised of the 'means of production' (i.e., land, animals, machines, which provide the resources for satisfying material human needs); 'the relations of production' (i.e., the power differential of one class over another) and 'means of consumption' (i.e., individual commodities consumed for subsistence or luxury). This characterization of production was developed in response to Georg Hegel's philosophical idealism (Hegel, 1977 [1807]; see also Giddens, 1971; Hughes et al., 2003).

In *The German Ideology* (Marx and Engels, 1947 [1845–7]), Marx proposed a framework to acknowledge the material world of human experience that prioritized questions of social existence and economic necessity. This differed from Hegel's focus on the material world as made known through human thought. For Marx, in his own words, 'life involves before everything eating, drinking, a habitation, clothing and many other things. The first act is thus the production of the means to satisfy these needs, the production of material life itself' (Marx and Engels, 1947

[1845–7]: 16). Morrison (2006) helpfully summarizes Marx's rejection of Hegel on four key premises. First, Marx asserted that human physical needs come before intellectual needs and physical, material needs can only be satisfied by direct productive activity – most simply, without a means of food and shelter, human beings cannot live. Second, the very real problems individuals face (i.e., the social conditions of the industrial worker and associated health consequences) are overlooked or ignored in favour of abstraction, thereby dissolving 'in the head' all the forces that limit human existence. Third, Marx rejected aspects of Hegel's framework whereby the realities of human hardship are theorized as historical actualities and inevitable processes, rather than individual acts that are endorsed by the state. Finally, in contrast to Hegel's assertion that individual freedom results from changes in individual consciousness, Marx thought that such a view amounts to asking individuals to interpret reality in a different way, when in fact they can only eliminate their hardship and social inequalities by altering their social and economic conditions.

It was in *The German Ideology* that Marx broke decisively with Hegel by developing the ideas of the German philosopher Ludwig Feuerbach and combining them with the socialist ideas of the French idealist Claude de Saint-Simon. Marx followed Feuerbach in inverting Hegel's notion of alienation, and extending it beyond considerations of religion, applying it most fervently in his analysis of economic production under capitalism. His adaptation of the alienation concept centres on issues of self-identity and human labour. Most simply it refers to the processes whereby the products of human labour become 'alien' to those who produce them (Lee and Newby, 1983), a paradox Marx took to be one of the central contradictions of capitalist society. In alienation's most developed form, the division of labour proceeds to a point where people are dominated by 'things', and market forces of production and consumption pervade every aspect of social life. Marx theorized ideology and contradiction as a means of understanding how social inequities (principally along the lines of social class divisions) come to exist side-by-side in society. Ideology is key to making inequalities appear legitimate and assigning their causes to sources other than social production (i.e., 'natural' laws and 'facts' of life). Marx believed that the inherent economic logic of capitalism (i.e., competition among capitalists; conflict between capital and labour) would ultimately lead to its collapse. As is evident in Chapter 2, modern history shows the opposite to be true – capitalism has intensified and diversified on a global scale. Arguably, that makes Marx's voluminous writings on capitalism more (rather than less) important as a basis for contemporary debate.[1]

The social relations of production and consumption

Marx was central in conceptualizing production and consumption as more than general economic categories universal across all societies.[2] His analysis of capitalism famously characterized it as a system of commodity production. In his words 'a commodity is, in the first place, an object outside of us, a thing that by its properties satisfies human wants of some sort or another' (Marx, 1976 [1867]: 13). His use of the phrase 'in the first *place*' is both intentional and important, as it alludes to the distinction between *use* value and *exchange* value. Most simply, use value refers to a commodity's ability to meet human needs, whereas exchange value is the exchange relation between one commodity and another. This point is key to understanding Marx's position on value as predominantly a product of social relations. Furthermore, his term 'commodity fetishism' articulates the process whereby a commodity is assigned extraordinary value and powers (giving the object a power akin to religious significance), which results in human relations to these objects becoming one of desire.[3] Most importantly, the power ascribed to these commodities is believed to be inherent in the object (as opposed to a product of human labour). It is through the process of commodity fetishism that humans form relations with objects that may surpass relations with each other. In other words, when social relations between people are converted into object relations between things, a commodity can 'assume a fantastic form different from its reality' (Marx, 1976 [1867]: 170). According to Marx, infinite consumption needs are unique to the capitalist mode of production.

While the consumption concept can be traced to nineteenth-century origins (Marx, 1971 [1876]; Veblen, 2005 [1899]), most commentators agree that it was not until the last decades of the twentieth century that it became fundamentally important to the social sciences. Its status as a key concern of contemporary sociology is in part attributable to suggestions that it epitomizes wider social change. According to Bocock (1993), in late twentieth-century forms of capitalism, the consumption concept became increasingly conceived more as a social and cultural process (involving cultural signs and symbols), and less as an economic one. This is evident in the sociologist Zygmunt Bauman's (2007) claim that consumption is a trait and occupation of individuals and consumerism is an attribute of society where 'consumption takes over that linchpin role which was played by work in the society of producers' (Bauman, 2007: 28). Yet, at the same time as this definition is offered, Bauman himself cautions against composing any cohesive view of consumers and their life strategies as new social hierarchies (based on possessions or adaptations of oneself) emerge. Similarly, as Brewer and Trentmann (2006: 13) highlight, in seeking to do justice to contemporary consumption 'no single narrative of consumption, no single typology of the consumer and no monolithic version of consumer culture will suffice'. The inadequacies of a single, static definition of consumption are evident in Jean Baudrillard's (1998 [1970]) evolving discussion of the processes and significations of consumption in *The Consumer Society: Myths and Structures*. Written from a Marxist perspective, it is widely criticized for its production bias and cynicism about consumption as an increasingly important social and cultural phenomenon. Having said that, it does offer production as a framework to generate debate about consumption.

Baudrillard conceived the consumption concept as a structure akin to a Durkheimian social fact (see Chapter 2), that is external to and coercive over individuals, where 'the system of needs is the product of the system of production' (Baudrillard, 1998 [1970]: 74). While for Marx the process of alienation was a key contradiction of capitalist society, Baudrillard asserts that the central contradiction of contemporary capitalism is potentially unlimited productivity (fuelled by technological development) and the need to dispose of these products. One consequence is that needs and consumption become the organized extension of the *forces of production*. Thus, the meaning ascribed to objects based on basic human need shifts from actual use-value to encompass sign-value. In his words 'the washing machine *serves* as an appliance and *acts* as an element of prestige, comfort etc. It is strictly the latter field that is the field of consumption' (Baudrillard, 1998 [1970]: 77, emphasis in original). As objects and needs become substitutable, a new unconscious social logic emerges whereby human needs become infinite, with the finest of all consumer objects being the human body. What is more, this framework, precisely because of its temporal connection, speaks to the theorizing of medicalization in the same era (discussed below). As Donna Haraway (1997) has since pointed out, Marx showed us how objects and their making (both their material reality and how they are known) are full of labour, which includes nature, health and what counts as enhancement in the zone of capitalist market relations. Political economy of health perspectives, theorizing on medicalization and, more recently, biomedicalization, all speak to precisely these points.

Application of the production concept in health and medicine

The growth of interest in medicine and health as topics of concern for the social sciences from the 1960s onwards saw a range of scholars developing the concept of production from orthodox Marxist approaches. One key approach this work gave rise to was a concerted focus on the political economy of health (e.g., Ginzberg, 1965; Ehrenreich and Ehrenreich, 1970; Kelman, 1971; Krause, 1971; Doyal and Pennell, 1979), which introduced the term 'Medical Industrial Complex' (Wohl, 1984; Mckinlay and Stoeckle, 1988). This concept emphasizes medicine and healthcare as multimillion-dollar industries where the pursuit of profit runs contrary to the pursuit of health. In particular, Barbara Ehrenreich and John Ehrenreich's (1970) analysis of the American healthcare system detailed linkages between scientific knowledge construction, which serves as a vehicle for the application of certain technologies, which in turn benefit big business alliances between medicine and industry. Industries that organize consumption according to production include 'corporations in the health business, medical research physicians, university medical-school teaching hospitals, the Federal government' (Krause, 1971: 52). Other authors have shown how medicine and science are ideological enterprises that follow the logic of exchange value (Navarro, 1976; Figlio, 1978) and that the capitalist mode of production creates ill health (Figlio, 1978; Doyal and Pennell, 1979). For example, industrial workers may 'suffer directly, either through industrial injuries and diseases, or in more diffuse ways with stress related ill-health or psychosomatic problems' (Doyal and Pennell, 1979: 25). They may also suffer *indirect* effects on health from the environmental damage associated with industrialized production.

Another key approach explored the relationship between medicine and capitalism by developing the production concept in relation to medicalization. During the 1960s and 1970s, medicalization was principally defined as a 'process whereby more and more of everyday life has come under medical dominion, influence and supervision' (Zola, 1983: 295). Among the early medicalization theorists (Szasz, 1963; Freidson, 1970; Zola, 1972; Conrad, 1975; Illich, 1975; Oakley, 1980), Ivan Illich was most vociferous in suggesting that medicalization is a by-product of industrialized society. In his words, 'over-medicalization is a particularly painful example of frustrating over-production' (Illich, 1975: 61). For Illich, the medical establishment is itself a major threat to health in the form of 'iatrogenesis' or, in other words, medically induced harm. His model of the preventable harm done by medicine had three tiers: the physical damage caused by doctors in their attempts to cure individuals (clinical iatrogenesis); the addiction of individuals to medical care as a solution to problems (social iatrogenesis); and the destruction of the patient's autonomy (structural iatrogenesis). Thus:

> Medical Nemesis is more than all clinical iatrogeneses put together, more than the sum of malpractice, negligence, professional callousness, political maldistribution, medically decreed disability and all the consequences of medical trial and error. It is the expropriation of man's coping ability by a maintenance service which keeps him geared up at the service of the industrial system.
>
> (Illich, 1975: 160)

In essence, Illich was talking about *how*, as industrial-medical markets increase, demand is created rather than acute needs met, where increased usage infers demand and health improvement, but paradoxically masks ineffectiveness and actual harm. Moreover, the application of the industrial engineering approach to medicine furthers the view of the body as a machine (see Chapter 7), with constituent parts to be checked, fixed or replaced entirely through, arguably unnecessary, medical intervention. 'The doctor's grasp over life starts with the monthly pre-natal check-up, when he decides if and how the foetus shall be born; it ends with his decision to abandon further resuscitation' (Illich, 1975: 44–45). Thus, it becomes possible to see the very specific ways medicalization serves to uphold and extend industrialism on an infinite scale, with over-medicalization increasingly creating medical consumers across the spectrum of human life and reproduction – a point taken up later in this chapter in relation to caesarean birth.

Early critiques of Illich were concerned with his exclusive focus on the negative effects of medicine, with no consideration of its beneficence (Strong, 1979), his anti-technology stance (Doyal and Pennell, 1979), and his inherent assumptions about industrialism, rather than the capitalist system's need to sustain a particular set of social and economic relationships within the spheres of production and consumption (Navarro, 1976). Vicente Navarro's four decades of theorizing on medicalization (Navarro, 1976, 1986, 1999, 2007) has served as an important rejoinder to Illich's work. In *Medicine Under Capitalism* (1976) he first challenged Illich's use of industrialism as the prevalent ideology to explain Western 'developed' societies, favouring instead a return to Marx and capitalism as the primary (although not exclusive) determinant of the social formation of society and the system of medicine. Most simply, Navarro (1976) contested Illich's (1975) suggestion that the root of iatrogenesis is medicine, contending instead that dependency and consumption of all that is medical is a symptom of the larger root cause: capitalism. In his words, medicine reinforces and 'capitalizes on what is *already* there – *the need for consumption*' (Navarro, 1976: 112, emphasis in original).

By the late 1980s, medical sociologists had begun to suggest that clinical medicine had been fundamentally transformed from its late eighteenth- and nineteenth-century form. Uta Gerhardt (1989) identifies the reasons for this shift as including: the decline of old infectious diseases; patient and consumer group challenges to medical paternalism; significantly rising costs without significant health gains; and individual health behaviours and lifestyle factors as the new targets for medicine. Adele Clarke and colleagues (2010) identify three distinct periods of transformation: first, the rise of medicine (1890–1945); second, the medicalization era (circa 1940–85); and third, the present period, which is characterized by biomedicalization (1985 onwards). Clarke et al. (2010) suggest a new biopolitical economy of medicine, health, illness, living and dying, to not only treat but to prevent diseases, manage risks and optimize health. If the medicalization era spawned the Medical Industrial Complex, for Clarke et al. (2010) the biomedicalization era is characterized by the Biomedical Technoscience Corporacomplex, Inc. – a term they use to emphasize the corporatized and privatized (rather than state-funded) nature of research, products and services made possible by techno-scientific innovations that further biomedicalization.[4] The co-constituted, overlapping key processes associated with biomedicalization are:

> major political economic shifts; a new focusing on health and risk surveillance biomedicines; the techno-scientization of biomedicine; transformations of the production, distribution, and consumption of biomedical knowledges; and transformations of bodies and identities.
>
> (Clarke et al., 2010: 57)

In the field of human reproduction, the terms 'fertility-industrial complex' (Spar, 2006) and 'Fertility, Inc.' (Mamo, 2010) are used to make comparable points.

Theorizing about medicalization in the twentieth century further emphasizes the increasing significance of transnational capitalism, consumer health movements and biomedical enhancements (Conrad, 2005, 2007). Biomedical enhancements take many forms, including surgery, pharmacology and genetic intervention (Conrad, 2007). Reproductive health is one area where interventions proliferate in ways that muddy the lines between treatment and enhancement. Human reproduction, and the female reproductive body in particular, provides an illustrative case study of the enduring relevance of the production concept *and* the value of the consumption concept as co-constitutive of contemporary reproductive choices and constraints.

The social relations of (re)production

'Labour', the kind that men (and women) do in return for a wage, and the social relations that stem from it, is an enduring concern of sociology, one that originates from Marx and Durkheim (see Chapter 2). The other kind of labour, that which only women can do, which involves gestating and bringing forth a child, has been enthusiastically taken up in feminist social science scholarship on human reproduction. Influenced by and in response to increasing male interest in the application of scientific principles to childbirth, scholarly concerns with reproduction, culture and society are evident in early feminist sociological (Wollstonecraft, 1792; Martineau, 2009 [1837]) and classical anthropological thought (Westermarck, 1921 [1891]). But it was during the 1970s and early 1980s that human reproduction became a substantive field for the social sciences in its own right.

Anthropologists Faye Ginsberg and Rayna Rapp (1995) identify several key trajectories through which both the study of reproduction emerged and reproduction and production have become increasingly bound up with each other. These trajectories include studies of the control of reproduction through population policy and international development initiatives, studies of the meaning of reproduction over the course of the lifecycle, and studies of the medicalization of reproduction and the emergence of new reproductive technologies (see Chapter 5). Shifts in late twentieth-century reproductive and foetal medicine saw low-tech options for assisted conception (artificial insemination and traditional surrogacy) joined with (if not displaced by) high-tech procedures (derivative of in vitro fertilization, IVF), alongside equally high-tech biomedical developments in the surveillance and management of pregnancy. Ellen Annandale (1998) identifies distinct sociological strands of investigation into reproduction that seek to illuminate women's health concerns (including the medicalization of pregnancy and childbirth, as well as maternity as a transition point in women's lives), to highlight the associations between gender and health, and to use reproduction to draw attention to wider concerns in society. Thus, during the 1970s and early 1980s, feminist theory literally turned attention 'from the social relations of production to the social relations of *re*production' (Annandale, 1998: 74, emphasis in original).

The anthropologist Emily Martin's (1987) study of menstruation, birth and the menopause, *The Woman in the Body*, was formative in exposing the social production of knowledge about reproduction (both the embodiment of knowledge and the context specificity of its production). Martin's critical reading of the construction of reproduction in medical literature was combined with women's detailed accounts of their reproductive experiences and showed that they are not fragmented from other aspects of their situation such as class and race. Her argument is a call for a more comprehensive way of conceiving reproduction than medical science alone can offer. She explains, 'when medical doctors describe the labour that women do in childbirth, their expectations centre on how labour of other kinds is organized in our society and how technology and machinery can be used to control those who labour' (Martin, 1987: 66).

Through Martin's analysis of the metaphors of production that inform medical descriptions of female bodies (particularly during labour and childbirth), she shows that medicine does not objectively describe scientific facts; it produces them. In so doing, science and medicine (re)produce patriarchal conceptions of labour insofar as the labour women perform for social reproduction in the home is devalued (with labour outside the home in the form of paid employment ascribed greater value and remuneration), *and* the labour women perform during childbirth in the hospital is judged principally in terms of machine production. In other words, the industrial capitalist form of social hierarchy and control is reproduced, with women as labourers and doctors as managers and with medical technologies developed in the pursuit of more efficient labour (women's and doctors'). On the one hand, Martin's (1987) critique of the medicalization of childbirth moved the notion of production from the division of labour in society to the control of women on hospital labour wards – a reading that has been taken up by midwives seeking to challenge this model of maternity care (Dykes, 2006; Walsh, 2006; Burns et al., 2012). On the other hand, it set the tone for a new generation of ethnographic studies that challenged the construction of women as passive in their engagement with reproduction.

Despite being the first and most abundantly studied topic in the feminist medicalization scholarship of the 1970s and 1980s, childbirth technologies have received comparatively little social science attention since. There are, however, many exemplars of studies of the newer reproductive technologies that take as their focus assisted conception (Franklin, 1997; Throsby, 2004; Thompson, 2005; Mamo, 2007), gestational surrogacy (Teman, 2010), reprogenetics (Franklin and Roberts, 2006) and antenatal screening (Rapp, 2000). As a result of anthropology, sociology and science and technology studies, there now exists a wealth of reproduction scholarship.[5] Collectively this work demonstrates the critical value of production in drawing together old questions about the relations of production with new questions about the commodification of childbirth and maternal choice. This is especially important as the evolving processes of medicalization coalesce with those of biomedicalization in women's pregnancy and birth trajectories.

(Re)production reconsidered: the making of planned caesarean birth

Childbirth is an everyday occurrence where calls for ever-greater reliance on technology are countered by proponents of minimal intervention (see Beckett, 2005; Brubaker and Dillaway, 2009). However, at the same time as technologies of uncertain clinical benefit may have become routinely used in practice (ultrasound scans, electronic foetal monitoring, induction of labour, caesarean section), they are also increasingly sought by women where the prevailing milieu (created by childbirth activists and neoliberalism since the early 1990s) is one of choice, self-enhancement and individual responsibility. In resource-rich settings the world over, against the backdrop of privatized services and a for-profit healthcare industry, women's choice is presumed to be a legitimate component of maternity care; this, in turn, has constituted new forms of labour (in both senses of the word). While few social scientists have attended to how medicalization may now be apparent in actual childbirths (Brubaker and Dillaway, 2009) there has been increasing interest in caesarean section and the suggestion that women may now be choosing caesarean birth (Béhague, 2002; Beckett, 2005; Bergeron, 2007; Bryant et al., 2007; Kingdon, 2007; Bourgeault et al., 2008; Hewer et al., 2009; Douche and Carryer, 2011; McAra-Couper et al., 2011; Sahlin et al., 2013).

Vaginal delivery and caesarean section are two fundamentally different birth methods that have coexisted since ancient times (Francome et al., 1993). Vaginal birth is a physiological process that culminates in either the spontaneous expulsion or the assisted extraction of the baby and the placenta from a woman's vagina. Caesarean birth is a surgical method of delivery, where an incision is made into the abdomen and uterus and the baby is delivered through the mother's abdominal wall. As the term implies, spontaneous vaginal birth can happen without medical assistance or intervention. It was during the period Clarke et al. (2010) identify as the rise of medicine (1890–1945) that caesarean sections were first performed with any frequency and on mothers and babies who were likely to both survive. In England in 1953, only 2 per cent of all births were performed by caesarean section (Macfarlane et al., 2000); by the end of the twentieth century this figure was 21.3 per cent (Thomas and Paranjothy, 2001). It was in the UK during the 1990s that the suggestion that planned caesarean section[6] may be a preferable alternative to planned vaginal birth first gained momentum (Kingdon, 2007). Katherine Beckett's (2005) review of contemporary feminism and the politics of childbirth in the United States identifies the two kinds of argument that made 'choosing caesarean' possible in resource-rich Anglo-American contexts. The first is medical science's claim that caesareans have become safer (particularly for babies, but also for mothers) and the risks of vaginal birth (for mothers and babies) have been underestimated; the second is clinicians' support for the position that women now have the right to choose caesarean section in the absence of a medical reason. This brings to the fore many of the issues and concerns raised in old and new feminist literatures on (re)production, choice, technology, medicalization and biomedicalization.

Caesarean section for non-medical reasons has been described as the quintessential example of the medicalization of childbirth in the twenty-first century because as a 'treatment' it is by definition unnecessary; the surgery is potentially harmful (for mother and baby) and it is costly to the wider community (Wagner, 2000). Resonant with 'older' medicalization arguments, Veronique Bergeron (2007), writing in a North American context, argues that the reasons why some women prefer caesarean over vaginal birth is they are constrained by medicine's dominant birthing ethos (that labour and vaginal birth is inherently flawed) and their socialization into a world where childbirth has to fit around capitalist productivity (caesareans can be scheduled within an hour, whereas labour and vaginal birth takes much longer), fashion imperatives, limited healthcare resources and malpractice insurance. Other studies too suggest that women's choices are strongly influenced and determined by social change (specifically the neoliberal expectation of choice); the gendering of women (as primarily sexual objects); values such as control, convenience and a quick fix; as well as the wider normalization of surgery for enhancement (McAra-Couper et al., 2011).

As illustrated in Figure 4.1, public debate about whether or not women should be able to choose planned caesarean section centres on a particular conception of heteronormative pregnant beauty and birth that represents the shift from caesarean technology's 'use value' (as a means of delivering the baby when maternal or foetal health is compromised) to encompass its value as an element of prestige for women – one associated with higher-quality care or part of an identity project as a sexually attractive partner. The zip signifies the surgeon's incision, the purported convenience and control, and the avoidance of vaginal trauma, which planned caesarean birth professes to offer pregnant women. Together this image and the text construct a relationship between high levels of medical intervention during childbirth and who is to blame for rising rates of caesarean section. Thus, it highlights an important point that feminist science and technologies scholarship on assisted reproduction articulates: the increasing role of the media in producing and sustaining the phenomenon of planned caesarean section for maternal request, as new patterns of medical knowledge consumption develop and reliance on medical technologies increases.

In their employment of the production conception in relation to childbirth, both Martin (1987) and Barbara Katz Rothman (1989) highlighted the increasing significance of caesarean birth in the United States. In Martin's words it 'requires the most management by doctors, the least labour by women and is seen as providing the best product: a perfect baby' (Martin, 1987: 64). More recent scholarship contends that the baby is not the only product in-the-making. In an Australian context, Joanne Bryant and colleagues (2007: 1195) have shown how on the one hand the rhetoric of 'neoliberalism accords women entitlement to consumption of birthing services, or the right to choose the services and commodities that best suit their desired birth experience', but on the other hand this same discourse produces the obligation for women to manage risk in ways that diminish the choices available to them. In Bryant's study, when women were presented with the information that caesarean birth was safer for their baby it became the *only* responsible choice in the pursuit of an identity as a 'good mother'.

My own work in the UK (Kingdon, 2007) highlights the importance of medical technology in how women come to know their baby during pregnancy (through ultrasound scan images and foetal heart-rate monitors). This leads to raised maternal expectations and greater reliance on medical knowledge about their baby's

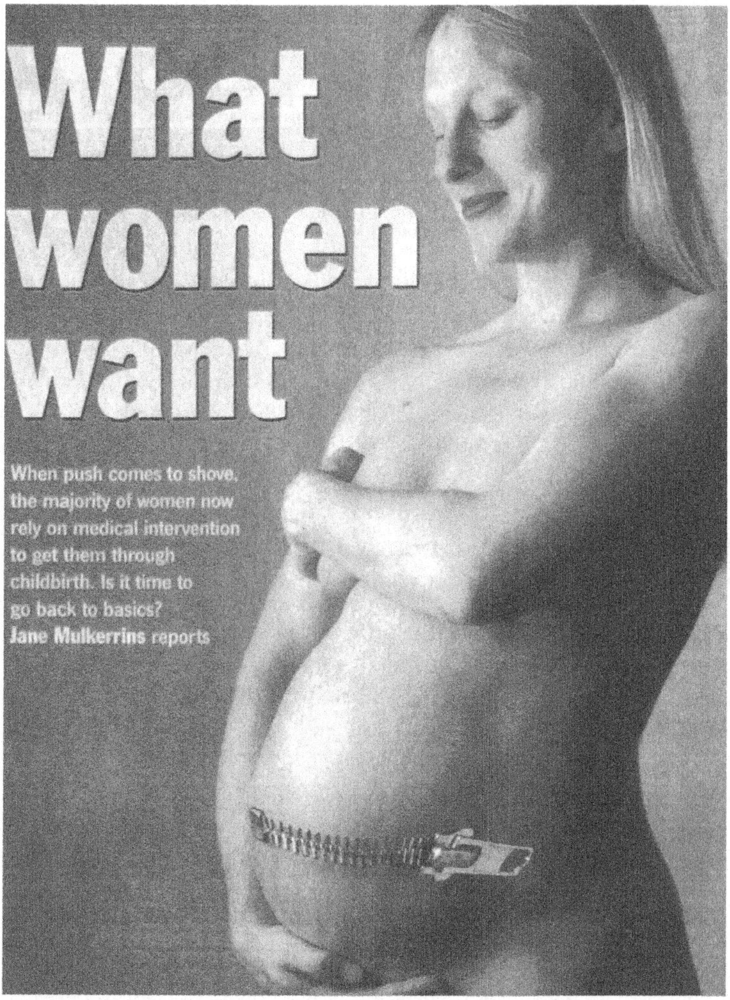

FIGURE 4.1 Cover of an article on the growing role of medical intervention in childbirth (Source: *The Sunday Times*, 2002, reproduced under licence).

safety, which limits their choice of birth method. The detailed accounts of women collected at three time-points during pregnancy and 12 months after birth also revealed knowledge acquisition about vaginal and caesarean birth to be a process where choice is fluid and only finite at actual delivery, thus challenging whether maternal choice for caesarean section really exists in the form assumed by much medical literature (Kingdon et al., 2009). Starting from pregnant women's vantage point, I showed that for many women choice is unstable, limited and undesirable, challenging the linear notion of choice that had hitherto dominated medical literature and practice guidelines. The situation of a particular group of women was highlighted in the relations between medical knowledge, everyday practices, material embodiment and technology, all of which are continuously co-constituted, and have world-making consequences (Kingdon, 2007).

The anthropologist Dominique Béhague (2002: 501) makes a similar point that caesarean birth as a concept and materiality is being continuously made with 'actual socio-clinical environments producing different kinds of births'. Focusing on the Brazilian context, Béhague (2002) moves beyond financial and physician-based explanations for rising caesarean section rates to show how planned caesarean section is associated with higher-quality care, and that particularly for some groups of women, it offers a route out of commonly experienced mistreatment and abuse during planned vaginal births. Béhague (2002) also makes the wider point that the current focus on whether the rise in caesarean births is driven by women or health professionals diverts attention away from how definitions of and indications for caesarean technology are themselves medically and socially altered(ing), which is in turn changing what is conceived as 'natural'.[7]

Between technology, doctors, patients and consumers: production and health in co-constituted futures

The linkages Ehrenreich and Ehrenreich (1970) first identified between scientific knowledge claims and the application of certain technologies that benefit big businesses, and the alliances between medicine and industry, have become more salient as biomedical knowledges, technologies, capitalism and consumerism become ever more intertwined (Haraway, 1997). Developments in reproductive genetics, assisted conception, pregnancy screening and labour surveillance both respond to and create demand for technological intervention, as do the relations between these technologies that give rise to raised maternal expectations (see Chapter 2). Early feminist medicalization scholarship drew attention to associations between induction of labour (which makes contractions more painful), epidurals (which numb the labour pain, but restrict mobility) and an increased likelihood of caesarean section (Cartwright, 1979; Oakley, 1980). There are now known associations between assisted conception, ultrasound scans, electronic foetal monitoring and caesarean section (planned and emergency).

There is also increasing evidence of rising rates of caesarean section in the private healthcare sector, although the extent to which is this attributable to planned caesarean section for non-medical reasons is debatable. Indeed, in Ireland the increased scheduling of planned caesarean section among private patients is creating new concerns about access issues for medically indicated caesareans (to finite theatre resources) and the disproportionate burden placed on postnatal health services (as caesarean births require post-operative care in addition to routine mother and baby care) (Murphy and Fahey, 2013).

For Illich (1975), medicalization was a by-product of industrialized society, a case of overproduction and the root of unnecessary harm. Planned caesarean section is one example of how, as the marketization of maternity care has increased, demand is created rather than acute needs met. The increased use of caesarean technology in itself infers greater demand and health improvement, but paradoxically masks the risks of the surgery, post-operative pain, and future morbidity and mortality (Lavender et al., 2012). Nevertheless, caesarean technology in specific circumstances is life-saving. In different circumstances, planned caesarean section for non-medical reasons may be considered 'life-enhancing' (Harer, 2000). Social scientists should no longer shy away from the biological conditions that produce the need for the technology, and stabilize and sustain its usage (Béhague, 2002). This is especially important as the consumer orientation in maternity care expands and childbearing women are constructed as consumers and patients.

Conclusion

In July 2013, the British newspaper *The Times* distributed a supplement focusing on private maternity care for expectant parents (*The Times*, 2013). The supplement included journalistic essays suggesting new demand for private maternity services, articles detailing clinician and celebrity endorsement accompanied by airbrushed images of mothers, babies and labour rooms styled like hotel suites, and direct-to-consumer advertisements from private healthcare providers. These included three of London's most prestigious National Health Service (NHS) Trusts, with one full-page advertisement using the headline 'Private caesarean sections at University College London Hospital'. Arguably, this single advertisement encapsulates both the transformation of the NHS in England (where the twin processes of deregulation and privatization now flourish) and exemplifies the global assumption in twenty-first-century maternity care that planned caesarean birth is a consumer choice. The emergence of consumers and new medical markets in present-day forms of Westernized neoliberal capitalism represents a significant change over the past 30 years, with these developments related, if not always explicitly connected (Conrad, 2007).

As the forces of transnational capitalism continue to redefine production and consumption in increasingly complex ways, this chapter has centred on women's reproductive health, with its inherent contradictions in health gains and health inequalities. A return to Marx has shown how fruitful his conception of the production concept is in thinking about contemporary developments in health, technology and medicine, which have in turn been taken up in formulations of political economy, medicalization, biomedicalization and feminist theorizing. This chapter has also shown that production has provided the grounding for rich feminist scholarship on reproduction and reproductive technologies (old and new), where it continues to prove fruitful in helping to understand how capitalism penetrates and transforms so-called 'natural' processes such as childbirth – an argument that is transferable to other areas of health, technology and medicine.

Notes

1 One important area where Marx's production concept has been taken up and further developed is feminist standpoint theory (Smith, 1987, 1990; Harding, 1991; Haraway, 1997). Dorothy Smith's variant of feminist standpoint theory argued that a focus on the material lives of women is less about a shift in subject matter for sociology and more (following Marx) about a different conception of sociology to understand both experience and the conditions of our experience (both women's and men's) in capitalist society. It is about who has the power over what is known and its world-making consequences.

2 The terms 'production' and 'consumption' were treated as purely economic categories up until the mid-nineteenth century.

3 For work that shows how 'commodity fetishism' has been taken up and worked through non-market societies, see Taussig (1980).

4 See Cooper (2008) and Rajan (2012) for further detail of the biotech industry, genomics and synthetic biology as new sites for the production of surplus.

5 Charis Thompson (2005) has usefully identified three chronological phases in feminist theorizing and research concerning assisted conception techniques that demonstrate the wealth of reproduction scholarship. The first phase, between 1984 and 1991, was when feminists first began to engage with the new reproductive technologies and many lines of argument were overtly critical. For example, some writers developed themes inherent in second-wave critiques of the medicalization of childbirth, others focused on the (in) equity of infertility treatment (along the lines of gender, class, race, age, able-bodiedness), while others concentrated on the ethical issues raised by these technologies. The second transition phase occurred between 1992 and 2000, when feminists began to move away from a 'just say no' approach to address the 'paradox of infertility'. For example, feminists began to undertake research addressing how these technologies raised issues for women at a structural level, while simultaneously offering real solutions for infertile women at the level of individual agency. It was also during this phase that a resurgence of interest in kinship emerged (see Chapter 5). The final phase, from 2000 to the present day, is characterized by a change in tone and focus, with current feminist writing on assisted conceptive techniques cautioning against simplistic readings of physicians and scientists (and women), often undertaken in clinical settings in collaboration with clinicians, and focusing on the active role of technology in shaping new and emerging relations of reproduction.

6 The term 'caesarean section' not only refers to the making of a surgical incision into the abdomen and uterus to deliver a baby through the mother's abdominal wall, it also encompasses many different degrees of urgency with which the operation may be performed dependent upon the rationale behind it that range from: acute medical need (immediately life-threatening), non-urgent medical need (scheduled for a medical reason), ambiguous medical need (failure to progress in labour or presumed foetal compromise) or non-medical reasons (increasingly categorized as maternal request). Caesarean delivery for maternal request has 'officially' been defined as a subset of elective (scheduled) caesarean delivery, performed not by medical necessity or indication, but on the request of the pregnant patient (National Institutes for Health, 2006).

7 See Chapter 5 for further discussion of the ways reproductive technologies transform notions of 'nature' and 'culture'.

References

Annandale, E. (1998) *The Sociology of Health and Medicine: A Critical Introduction*. Cambridge: Polity Press.

Baudrillard, J. (1998 [1970]) *The Consumer Society: Myths and Structures*. London: Sage.

Bauman, Z. (2007) *Consuming Life*. Cambridge: Polity Press.

Béhague, D. (2002) Beyond the simple economics of cesarean section birthing: women's resistance to social inequality. *Culture, Medicine and Psychiatry*, 26: 473–507.

Beckett, K. (2005) Choosing cesarean: feminism and the politics of childbirth in the United States. *Feminist Theory*, 6(3): 251–275.

Bergeron, V. (2007) The ethics of cesarean section on maternal request: a feminist critique of the American College of Obstetricians and Gynecologists' position on patient-choice surgery. *Bioethics*, 21(9): 478–487.

Bocock, R. (1993) *Consumption*. London: Routledge.

Bourgeault, I.V., Declerq, E., Sandall, J., Wrede, A. Vanstone, M., van Teijlingen, E., De Vries, R. and Benoit, C. (2008) Too posh to push? Comparative perspectives on maternal request caesarean sections in Canada, the US, the UK and Finland. *Patients, Consumers and Civil Society Advances in Medical Sociology*, 10: 99–123.

Brewer, J. and Trentmann, F. (eds.) (2006) *Consuming Cultures, Global Perspectives: Historical Trajectories, Transnational Exchanges*. London: Bloomsbury.

Brubaker, S.J. and Dillaway, H.E. (2009) Medicalization, natural childbirth and birthing experiences. *Sociology Compass*, 3: 31–48.

Bryant, J., Porter, M., Tracey, S.K. and Sullivan, E.A. (2007) Caesarean birth: consumption, safety, ordering and good mothering. *Social Science and Medicine*, 65: 1192–1201.

Burns, E., Schmied, V., Fenwick, J. and Sheehan, A. (2012) Liquid gold from the milk bar: constructions of breast milk and breastfeeding women in the language and practices of midwives. *Social Science and Medicine*, 75(10): 1737–1745.

Cartwright, A. (1979) *The Dignity of Labour? A Study of Childbearing and Induction*. London: Tavistock.

Clarke, A.E., Mamo, L., Fosket, J.R., Fishman, J.R. and Shim, J.K. (eds.) (2010) *Biomedicalization: Technoscience, Health and Illness in the US*. Durham, NC: Duke University Press.

Conrad, P. (1975) The discovery of hyperkinesis: notes on the medicalization of deviant behaviour. *Social Problems*, 23(1): 12–21.

Conrad, P. (2005) The shifting engines of medicalization. *Journal of Health and Social Behaviour*, 26(1): 3–14.

Conrad, P. (2007) *The Medicalization of Society: On the Transformation of Human Conditions Into Treatable Disorders*. Baltimore: Johns Hopkins University Press.

Cooper, M. (2008) *Life as Surplus: Biotechnology and Capitalism in the Neoliberal Era*. Seattle, WA: University of Washington Press.

Douche, J. and Carryer, J. (2011) Caesarean section in the absence of need: a pathologising paradox for public health? *Nursing Inquiry*, 18(2): 143–153.

Doyal, L. and Pennell, I. (1979) *The Political Economy of Health*. London: Pluto Press.

Dykes, F. (2006) *Breastfeeding in Hospital: Mothers, Midwives and the Production Line*. London: Routledge.

Ehrenreich, B. and Ehrenreich, J. (1970) *The American Health Empire: Power, Profits and Politics*. New York: Random House.

Figlio, K.M. (1978) Chlorosis and chronic disease in nineteenth-century Britain: the social constitution of somatic illness in a capitalist society. *Social History*, 3: 167–197.

Francome, C., Savage, W. and Churchill, H. (1993) *Caesarean Birth in Britain: A Book for Health Professionals and Parents*. London: Middlesex University Press.

Franklin, S. (1997) *Embodied Progress: A Cultural Account of Assisted Conception*. London: Routledge.

Franklin, S. and Roberts, C. (2006) *Born and Made: An Ethnography of Preimplantation Genetic Diagnosis*. Princeton, NJ: Princeton University Press.

Freidson, E. (1970) *Profession of Medicine: A Study of the Sociology of Applied Knowledge.* New York: Harper and Row.

Gerhardt, U. (1989) *Ideas About Illness: An Intellectual and Political History of Medical Sociology.* Basingstoke: Macmillan.

Giddens, A. (1971) *Capitalism and Modern Social Theory.* Cambridge: Cambridge University Press.

Ginsberg, F. and Rapp, R. (1995) *Conceiving the New World Order: The Global Politics of Reproduction.* Berkeley, CA: University of California Press.

Ginzberg, E. (1965) The political economy of health. *Bulletin of the New York Academy of Medicine,* 41: 1015–1036.

Haraway, D. (1997) *Modest_Witness@Second_Millenium. FemaleMan© Meets OncoMouse™: Feminism and Technoscience.* New York: Routledge.

Harding, S. (1991) *Whose Science? Whose Knowledge? Thinking from Women's Lives.* New York: Cornell University Press.

Harer, W. (2000) Patient choice cesarean. *ACOG Clinical Review,* 5: 1–15.

Hegel, G.W.F. (1977 [1807]) *Phenomenology of Spirit.* Oxford: Clarendon Press.

Hewer, N., Boschma, G. and Hall, W.A. (2009) Elective caesarean section as a transformative technological process: players, power and context. *Journal of Advanced Nursing,* 65(8): 1762–1771.

Hughes, J.A., Sharrock, W.W. and Martin, P.J. (2003) *Understanding Classical Sociology.* London: Sage.

Illich, I. (1975) *Medical Nemesis: The Expropriation of Health.* Great Britain: Calder & Boyars.

Kelman, S. (1971) Toward the political economy of medical care. *Inquiry,* 8: 30–38.

Kingdon, C. (2007) *Re-visioning Choice Through Situated Knowledges: Women's Preferences for Vaginal or Caesarean Birth.* Doctoral Dissertation. Department of Sociology, Lancaster University.

Kingdon, C., Neilson, J., Singleton, V., Gyte, G., Hart, A., Gabbay, M. and Lavender, T. (2009) Choice and birth method: mixed method study of caesarean delivery for maternal request. *BJOG: An International Journal of Obstetrics and Gynaecology,* 116(7): 886–895.

Krause, E. (1971) Health and the politics of technology. *Inquiry,* 8: 51–59.

Lavender, T., Hofmeyr, G.J., Neilson, J.P., Kingdon, C. and Gyte, G.M.L. (2012) Caesarean section for non-medical reasons at term. *Cochrane Database of Systematic Reviews,* 3: Art. No. CD004660.

Lee, D. and Newby, H. (1983) *The Problem of Sociology.* London: Unwin Hyman.

Macfarlane, A., Mugford, M. and Henderson, J. (2000) *Birth Counts: Statistics of Pregnancy and Childbirth,* Vol. 2. London: Stationery Office.

Mamo, L. (2007) *Queering Reproduction: Achieving Pregnancy in the Age of Technoscience.* Durham, NC: Duke University Press.

Mamo, L. (2010) Fertility Inc.: Consumption and subjectification in US lesbian reproductive practices. In A.E. Clarke, L. Mamo, J.R. Fosket, J.R. Fishman and J.K. Shim (eds.), *Biomedicalization: Technoscience, Health and Illness in the US.* Durham: Duke University Press, 173–196.

Martin, E. (1987) *The Woman in the Body.* Milton Keynes: Open University Press.

Martineau, H. (2009 [1837]) *Society in America.* Cambridge: Cambridge University Press.

Marx, K. (1971 [1876]) *Capital: A Critique of Political Economy,* Vol. 2. Moscow: Progress.

Marx, K. (1976 [1867]) *Capital: A Critique of Political Economy,* Vol. 1. Middlesex: Penguin.

Marx, K. (1977 [1859]) *A Contribution to the Critique of Political Economy.* Moscow: Progress Publishers.

Marx, K. and Engels, F. (1947 [1845–1847]) *The German Ideology.* New York: International Publishing.

McAra-Couper, J., Jones, M., and Smythe, L. (2011) Caesarean-section, my body, my choice: the construction of 'informed choice' in relation to intervention in childbirth. *Feminism and Psychology*, 22(1): 81–97.

McKinlay, J.B. and Stoeckle, J.D. (1988) Corporatization and the social transformation of doctoring. *International Journal of Health Services*, 18: 191–205.

Morrison, K. (2006) *Marx, Durkheim, Weber: Formations of Modern Social Thought*. London: Sage.

Murphy, D.J. and Fahey, T. (2013) A retrospective cohort study of mode of delivery among public and private patients in an integrated maternity hospital setting. *BMJ Open*, 3.

National Institutes for Health (2006) *Caesarean Delivery on Request: Final Panel Statement*. Available at: http://consensus.nih.gov/2006/cesareanstatement.htm#q4.

Navarro, V. (1976) *Medicine Under Capitalism*. New York: Prodist.

Navarro, V. (1986) *Crisis, Health, and Medicine: a Social Critique*. New York: Tavistock.

Navarro, V. (1999) Health and equity in the world in the era of globalization. *International Journal of Health Services*, 29(2): 215–226.

Navarro, V. (2007) *Neoliberalism, Globalization, and Inequalities: Consequences for Health and Quality of Life*. New York: Baywood.

Oakley, A. (1980) *Women Confined: Towards a Sociology of Childbirth*. Oxford: Martin Robertson.

Rajan, K.S. (ed) (2012) *Lively Capital: Biotechnologies, Ethics, and Governance in Global Markets*. Durham, NC: Duke University Press.

Rapp, R. (2000) *Testing Women, Testing the Fetus: The Social Impact of Amniocentesis in America*. New York: Routledge.

Rothman, B.K. (1989) *Recreating Motherhood: Ideology and Technology in a Patriarchal Society*. New York: W.W. Norton.

Sahlin, M., Carlander-Klint, A.K., Hildingsson, I. and Wiklund, I. (2013) First-time mothers' wish for a planned caesarean section: deeply rooted emotions. *Midwifery*, 29: 447–452.

Smith, D. (1987) *The Everyday World as Problematic: A Feminist Sociology*. Boston, MA: Northeastern University Press.

Smith, D. (1990) *The Conceptual Practices of Power*. Boston, MA: Northeastern University Press.

Spar, D.L. (2006) *The Baby Business: How Money, Science, and Politics Drive the Commerce of Conception*. Cambridge, MA: Harvard Business Review Press.

Strong, P. (1979) Sociological imperialism and the profession of medicine: a critical examination of the thesis of medical imperialism. *Social Science and Medicine*, 13A: 199–215.

Szasz, T.S. (1963) *Law, Liberty, and Psychiatry: An Inquiry into the Uses of Mental Health Practices*. New York: Macmillan.

Taussig, M. (1980) *The Devil and Commodity Fetishism*. Charlotte, NC: University of North Carolina Press.

Teman, E. (2010) *Birthing a Mother: The Surrogate Body and the Pregnant Self*. Berkeley, CA: University of California Press.

Thomas, J. and Paranjothy, S. (2001) *The National Sentinel Caesarean Section Audit Report*. London: RCOG Press.

Thompson, C. (2005) *Making Parents: The Ontological Choreography of Reproductive Technologies*. Cambridge, MA: MIT Press.

Throsby, K. (2004) *When IVF Fails: Feminism, Infertility and the Negotiation of Normality*. Basingstoke: Palgrave Macmillan.

The Times (2013) Report: private maternity. *Raconteur*. Available at: http://raconteur.net/private-maternity.

Veblen, T. (2005 [1899]) *Conspicuous Consumption: Unproductive Consumption of Goods is Honourable*. London: Penguin.

Wagner, M. (2000) Choosing caesarean section. *Lancet*, 356: 1677–1680.

Walsh, D. (2006) Subverting the assembly-line: childbirth in a free-standing birth centre. *Social Science and Medicine*, 62: 1330–1340.

Westermarck, E. (1921 [1891]) *The History of Human Marriage*. London: Macmillan.

Wohl, S. (1984) *The Medical Industrial Complex*. New York: Harmony.

Wollstonecraft, M. (1792) *Vindication of the Rights of Woman*. London: Joseph Johnson.

World Bank (2014) Health expenditure, total (% of GDP). Available at: http://data.worldbank.org/indicator/SH.XPD.TOTL.ZS.

Zola, I.K. (1972) Medicine as an institution of social control. *Sociological Review*, 20: 487–503.

Zola, I.K. (1983) *Socio-Medical Inquiries: Recollections, Reflections, and Reconsiderations*. Philadelphia, PA: Temple University Press.

5

KINSHIP

Kirsten Bell

> Interrogating kinship… continues to precipitate lively debate concerning not only what kinship is 'all about' but also how its uses index wider changes within anthropology as well as within the societies of which anthropologists are a part.
>
> Sarah Franklin and Susan McKinnon, *Relative Values: Reconfiguring Kinship Studies*

Introduction

In 1967, Robin Fox famously observed that 'kinship is to anthropology what logic is to philosophy or the nude is to art; it is the basic discipline of the subject' (Fox, 1967: 10). This statement has been so often reproduced not because of its incisiveness or accuracy, but because less than 15 years after Fox wrote it, it seemed so hopelessly antiquated. By this stage, there had been a clear turn away from the topic of kinship in the discipline, which had become distinctly unfashionable as a subject matter. While earlier generations of anthropologists prioritized the study of kinship to such a degree that they often bribed and cajoled recalcitrant informants to obtain this information,[1] many anthropologists today (myself included) would be hard-pressed to draw a kinship diagram, such graphical depictions of kin relations being deemed useful fodder for first-year lectures but not much else. And yet, interest in kinship, as many commentators have observed, has undergone something of a resurgence in recent years.

In this chapter I do not seek to perpetuate the idea that the study of kinship in anthropology essentially died out, only to re-emerge like a phoenix rising from the ashes. As Sarah Franklin and Susan McKinnon (2001: 6) observe: 'Kinship study has not reawakened, like some disciplinary Sleeping Beauty waiting to be rescued;

rather, it has been steadily reinventing itself and, in the process, has undergone a substantial makeover.' However, while the study of kinship never disappeared entirely, its central concerns have undergone a radical reconfiguration over the past 40-odd years, much in tandem with larger transformations in the discipline, as outlined in the discussion of culture in Chapter 1.

In what follows, I intend to trace some of these reconfigurations of kinship. In light of the ways that anthropologists staked such a claim over the concept, the overview of its history is weighted heavily towards anthropological scholarship. However, I do *not* intend to 'excavate particular histories of the anthropological kinship theory' (Edwards, 2009: 2) – a task that others have accomplished far more ably than I could hope to attempt in the space of a chapter (see Peletz, 1995; Holy, 1996; Franklin and McKinnon, 2001; Carsten, 2004).[2] I aim to show the ways that discussions about kinship have illuminated the relationship between nature and culture – or, more accurately, challenged the distinction itself and the assumption that the appropriate object of anthropological work is the 'social' aspects of kinship, with the 'biological' hived off as both primordial and pre-given. To this end, I begin with an overview of the predominant ways kinship has been conceptualized in anthropology, paying particular attention to the internal critiques that have always been a part of the field (and historically accounted for much of its vibrancy). I then explore the state of kinship studies today, which is flourishing across the social sciences, focusing especially on the impact of new reproductive and genetic technologies in the reconfiguration of the topic. Finally, in an effort to empirically ground and pull together the various strands developed in the chapter, I focus on contemporary enactments of kinship in the context of genetic cancer counselling.

A social elaboration of natural facts: early approaches to kinship

From anthropology's inception, the study of kinship was deemed a central concern of the discipline because it was a category that seemed to be simultaneously biological *and* social – 'a special instance of the general manner in which human beings construct societies and cultures "out of" nature' (Strathern, 1992a: 4). Although conventional scientific thinking suggested that kinship was a 'fact of nature', anthropologists insisted that it was a 'cultural and not merely a natural fact' (Malinowski, 1930: 24). Anthropologists observed that although all societies recognized some form of kinship, they differed dramatically in the ways they organized it, perhaps best illustrated through Bronisław Malinowski's (1929) writing on the variable character of the incest taboo. In Fox's words:

> Kinship and marriage are about the basic facts of life… Although Man has these facts of life in common with other mammals, he differs in that he can choose between the alternative courses that they offer him in the way of group-formation, succession, mating arrangements, etc. His choice is often

> constrained within narrow limits but the fact remains that he can *do* things with the basic bonds arising from the processes of mating, childbearing, and childrearing.
>
> (Fox, 1967: 1, emphasis in original)

The topic therefore generated considerable excitement for early anthropologists, with the work of Lewis Henry Morgan instrumental in developing (or 'inventing') kinship studies[3] (see Trautman, 1987). It was Morgan who established what later became the central preoccupations of the field, including the emphasis on biological relations among people as the basis for ordering their social relations and his focus on kinship terminologies as the key to understanding folk models of biological consanguinity – and their historic origins (see Holy, 1996 for further discussion). In his *Ancient Society: Researches in the Lines of Human Progress From Savagery Through Barbarism to Civilization*, Morgan (1985 [1877]) traced the progression of the family from an initial stage of 'promiscuous intercourse', through to the 'monogamian family' (stage V). Along the lines of Edward Tylor's evolutionary model of culture (see Chapter 1), the kinship institutions of 'primitive' peoples were seen to provide insights into earlier stages of cultural evolution, which were in turn traced back to hypothesized antecedents.

If Morgan helped to established kinship as a domain of anthropological import, it was the work of W.H.R. Rivers, in particular his genealogical method, that provided fieldworkers with their key toolkit for studying it. Based on work in the Torres Strait, Rivers (1900, 1910) highlighted the value of collecting detailed genealogical information from native informants as a means of studying larger sociological questions. In his words,

> I soon found that the knowledge possessed by the natives of their families was so extensive, and apparently so accurate, that a complete collection of the genealogies as far back as they could be traced would be interesting and might enable one to study many sociological problems more exactly than would be otherwise possible.
>
> (Rivers, 1900: 74)

Although Rivers' genealogical method had a profound influence on British social anthropology, Morgan's work (and Rivers' to a lesser extent) was criticized by key figures such as A.R. Radcliffe-Brown. Of Morgan's work, Radcliffe-Brown spoke disparagingly of 'pseudo-historical' theories of kinship, whereby:

> starting from some known condition in the present or in the historically recorded past, an 'explanation' of it is invented by imagining some condition or event in the unrecorded past and arguing on *a priori* grounds that the known condition might or must have had its origin in this way.
>
> (Radcliffe-Brown, 1950: 1)

Targeting Rivers as well as Morgan, he also argued that the allegiance to pet theories had blinded scholars to the 'facts' of kinship on the ground, leading them 'into confusion that they might have avoided if it had not been present in their minds, influencing their assumptions and their observation'[4] (Radcliffe-Brown, 1929: 51).

Others – most prominently Malinowski – bemoaned what they saw as the highly esoteric atmosphere pervading kinship studies, and the obsession with long lists of native words, dry and complicated diagrams and formulae and so on, which served to alienate all but a few intrepid souls. In his words,

> The average anthropologist... somewhat mystified and perhaps a little hostile, has remained outside the narrow ring of devotees. He has his doubts whether the effort needed to master the bastard algebra of kinship is really worth while. He feels, that, after all, kinship is a matter of flesh and blood, the result of sexual passion and maternal affection, of long intimate daily life, and of a host of personal intimate interests.
>
> (Malinowski, 1930: 19)

What is striking about both Radcliffe-Brown and Malinowski's criticisms is the way they prefigured later critiques of kinship studies, a point to which I will return below. However, unlike the later reassessments, the goal of such commentaries was to improve the study of kinship as opposed to challenging some of its fundamental tenets.

For British social anthropologists, comparison and analysis of existing kinship systems remained a key priority for decades to follow. As Janet Carsten (2004) observes, these figures saw kinship – in the form of unilineal descent groups[5] and their formations as lineages and clans – as modes of organization that were central to the political structure and social continuity of stateless societies. E.E. Evans-Pritchard's (1940) work on the political institutions of the Nuer was seen to be exemplary in this regard. He described a 'segmentary lineage' political system based on principles of autonomous organization and inter-tribal affiliation or opposition. In the system he outlined, tribes were divided into segments, which were themselves further divided and so on, with segments only emerging as units of action as specific situations (most commonly fighting) demanded. Thus, depending on the context, segments would expand or contract (see Figure 5.1). In Evans-Pritchard's words, 'when Z^1 fights Z^2 no other section is involved. When Z^1 fights Y^1, Z^1 and Z^2 unite as Y^2. When Y^1 fights X^1, Y^1 and Y^2 unite, and so do X^1 and X^2. When X^1 fights A, X^1, X^2, Y^1, and Y^2 all unite as B' (1940: 143–144).

However, evident in Evans-Pritchard's work was some awareness of the artificiality of the system he outlined from the Nuer point of view. He observed in passing:

> A Nuer rarely talks about his lineage as distinct from his community, and in contrast to other lineages which form part of it, outside a ceremonial context. I have watched a Nuer who knew precisely what I wanted, trying on

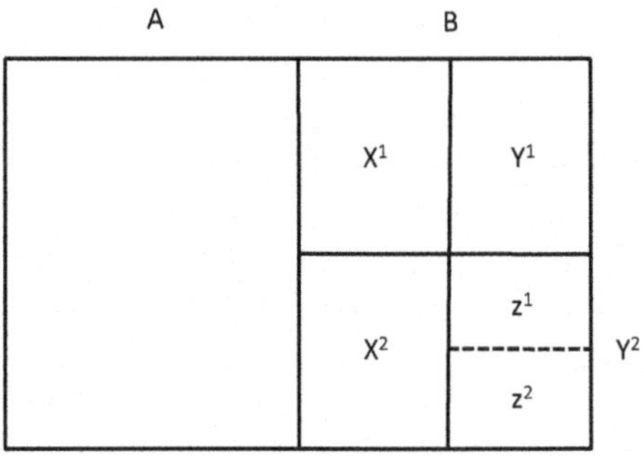

FIGURE 5.1 The Nuer segmentary lineage (adapted from Evans-Pritchard, 1940).

> my behalf to discover from a stranger the name of his lineage. He often found great initial difficulty in making the man understand the information required of him, for Nuer think generally in terms of local divisions and the relations between them, and an attempt to discover lineage affiliations apart from their community relations, and outside a ceremonial context, generally led to misunderstanding in the opening stages of an inquiry.
>
> (Evans-Pritchard, 1940: 203)

This difficulty of disentangling kinship from other domains (and the problems resulting from the efforts to isolate it) was to become a prominent theme in the later efforts to rethink the concept.

The dominant structural functionalist approaches to kinship were challenged by the emergence of French structuralism (see Chapter 1). The differences between the British and French schools of thought on kinship have been comprehensively documented in the work of Louis Dumont (2006 [1971]) so I won't dwell on them here, other than to say that Lévi-Strauss's approach was instrumental in expanding the focus of kinship studies from consanguineal ('blood') relationships to affinal (marital) ones. Highlighting the universality of the incest taboo, Lévi-Strauss derided explanations that treated the prohibition as stemming from natural causes or cultural conditions. In his words,

> The prohibition of incest is in origin neither purely cultural nor purely natural, nor is it a composite mixture of elements from both nature and culture. It is the fundamental step because of which, by which, but above all in which, the transition from nature to culture is accomplished.
>
> (Lévi-Strauss, 1969: 24)

Lévi-Strauss stressed the role of the incest taboo in ensuring exogamy, which in turn generated exchange between groups;[6] through marriage, men exchanged women, the 'supreme gift' (Carsten, 2004: 13).

As Carsten (2004) observes, although many were suspicious of the general structuralist tendency to understand culture in terms of paired oppositions (nature/culture, female/male and so on),[7] subsequent kinship scholars could not ignore Lévi-Strauss's insights regarding marriage as a long-term exchange involving the transfer of people, goods and services that cemented relations between two groups of affines. She also points out that despite the clear differences between structuralist-functionalist and structuralist approaches to kinship, they shared an emphasis on normative kinship roles and their underlying assumptions about the role (and nature) of women.

The critique of kinship coalesces

According to Ladislav Holy (1996), by the middle of the twentieth century, kinship studies constituted approximately half of the total anthropological literature. However, kinship as a distinct sub-discipline of anthropology became increasingly marginal throughout the 1970s and 1980s (Carsten, 2004). David Schneider's (1984) *A Critique of the Study of Kinship* is generally deemed to be instrumental in dismantling kinship as a separate domain of inquiry. In a trenchant critique of the epistemological problems with the concept, Schneider argued that what previous scholars had reported as the kinship systems of the people they studied were largely a result of their own theoretical apparatuses, as opposed to actually representing what they claimed to be: ethnographic facts. In particular, he described two key assumptions in prevailing theories of kinship: the 'doctrine of the genealogical unity of mankind', with its implication that genealogical relations are the same everywhere, and 'the assumption that blood is thicker than water', with its implication that genealogical bonds are unique (Schneider, 1984: 174; Franklin and McKinnon, 2001: 2). Drawing impetus from his earlier work *American Kinship: A Cultural Account* (Schneider, 1980 [1968]), Schneider argued that these assumptions were based on folk models of kinship derived from anthropologists' own cultures, which formulated kinship ties in biogenetic terms.

The persuasiveness of Schneider's argument rested on his analysis of his own fieldwork data among the Yapese from Micronesia, in which he produced two contrasting descriptions of kinship using different conceptual frames. His deconstructive efforts showed that this 'thing' called kinship was essentially an artefact of anthropological theories. In other words, such theories actively produced the very thing they aimed to describe. Schneider's critique exemplified a broader shift in anthropology in the 1970s and 1980s towards more self-critical and reflexive approaches (Franklin and McKinnon, 2001). The book's emphasis on the ways anthropological kinship theories imposed Western ontologies on non-Western peoples reflected the larger postcolonial and postmodern turn in anthropology, which saw the discipline's other foundational concepts undergo a similar shakedown, such as culture (see Chapter 1).

However, although the interrogations of kinship studies reached their climax in the 1980s, as previously indicated, earlier scholars – including the chief architects of functionalist and structural functionalist approaches – were not unaware of the problems with the field. They too highlighted the dry formalism of predominant theories and their inability to grasp the 'flesh and blood' of kinship relations, the role of anthropological classifications in producing what they aimed to study, and the resulting disconnect between anthropological and indigenous categories. Moreover, these criticisms continued apace into the 1950s, 1960s and 1970s. For example, Edmund Leach's *Rethinking Anthropology* highlighted the tautological dimensions of various studies of descent systems, where 'the system of classification already implies the truth of what she [the anthropologist] claims to be demonstrating' (Leach, 1961: 4). Likewise, Rodney Needham's edited volume *Rethinking Kinship and Marriage* emphasized the need to rely more on indigenous conceptions and categories and less on conventional typological guidelines and the 'false principles and false categories' (Needham, 1971: xx) they had produced.

Although Schneider's work introduced a wholesale questioning of what was 'natural' about kinship, as Franklin and McKinnon (2001) discuss, his identification of kinship as a primary site of anthropology's biologistic and Eurocentric tendencies echoed points made from the 1970s by feminist anthropologists (see Rosaldo and Lamphere, 1974; MacCormack and Strathern, 1980).[8] Such feminist critiques of kinship reached their epitome in Jane Collier and Sylvia Yanagisako's (1987) edited volume *Gender and Kinship: Essays Toward a Unified Analysis*. In this book, contributors challenged the traditional analytical boundary between gender and kinship as distinct domains of analysis and the attendant opposition between the domestic and politico-jural (public) spheres, arguing that these domains were mutually constituted. Collier and Yanagisako pointed out that in the analysis of both gender and kinship, anthropologists had made a similar error: taking for granted what needed to be explained (Carsten, 2004). In their words:

> Our critical review of the analytical dichotomies informing gender studies leads us to conclude that they, like the concepts informing kinship studies, assume the biological difference in male and female roles in sexual reproduction to be at the core of men's and women's relationships everywhere. We argue that, as a consequence, what have been conceptualized as two discrete fields of study constitute a single field defined by our folk conception of the same thing, namely, the biological facts of sexual reproduction.
>
> (Collier and Yanagisako, 1987: 7)

This emphasis on the mutual imbrication of gender and kinship served to upset the distinction between sex and gender and reproduction and kinship as 'natural' and 'cultural' categories respectively (Carsten, 2004)[9] – insights that had important implications for scholarship on the body more broadly (see Chapter 7 for further discussion).

'After nature':[10] kinship studies today

The analysis of processes of 'naturalization' in conceptions of kinship was extended in the work of Marilyn Strathern, which proved foundational for much contemporary scholarship on the topic (Franklin and McKinnon, 2001). As Franklin and McKinnon (2001) observe, Strathern's (1992a, 1992b) accounts of kinship reconfigured the critique of nature and natural facts as an examination of knowledge production more broadly. Through an ambitious, synthetic examination of English kinship constructs and her work on the new reproductive technologies, Strathern convincingly showed that nature has lost its grounding function as a condition for knowledge. Although it retains its salience as an organizing concept, 'what is taken to be natural has itself become a matter of choice' (Carsten, 2004: 167). This destabilization of the capacity for nature to be seen as a separate and distinct domain is particularly evident in the realm of new reproductive technologies. In Strathern's words:

> Contemporary possibilities of artificial procreation introduce a new contrast between artificial and natural process: assisted reproduction creates the biological parent as a separate category. By the same process, the social parent becomes marked as potentially deficient in biological credentials... So the 'natural' parent of the future, if one may extrapolate, may well turn out to be the one for whom no special legislation is required. In that case it would be the natural parent who combined both biological and social/legal attributes.
> (Strathern, 1992b: 20)

New reproductive technologies proved so 'good to think' with, for some, their emergence was pivotal in 'making kinship relevant again' (Parkin, 2006: ix; see also Peletz, 1995; Carsten, 2004), although their effects were also felt well beyond the realm of kinship studies – as Chapter 4 attests. As Franklin and McKinnon (2001) highlight, studies of adoption, surrogacy, in vitro fertilization (IVF) and so on, along with research on gay and lesbian kinship, have shown how the category of kinship may be conceived outside of its 'ruling sign of biology' (2001: 6). For example, Franklin's (1997) study of women and couples undergoing IVF in England illustrated the ways in which assisted reproduction troubled previous certainties regarding the 'genealogical grid that was once assumed to be both primordial, "rimless" and irrevocable' (1997: 8). The disquiet such technologies caused was evident in the 1990 Human Fertilization and Embryology Act and the debates it generated about conception, paternity and maternity, and other so-called 'facts of life'.[11]

However, for all the malleability such technologies were perceived to introduce, the concept of 'nature' was still central to popular and medical discourses on their utilization. Such accounts reveal the way in which nature has become technologized and technology has become naturalized, with what is attributable to 'nature' and to 'technology' increasingly blurred (Franklin, 1997; Carsten, 2004). Thus, IVF was often conceptualized as 'giving nature a helping hand', and the desire for treatment was framed in terms of the 'primordial' drive to reproduce (Franklin, 1997: 200). However, according to Franklin, assisted reproduction simultaneously served to increase rather than reduce the opacity of conception – especially given the high failure rates of IVF, writ in the lexicon of IVF technicians as 'unexplained infertility' (1997: 200). Her work also showed the interchanges between state and individual perspectives on assisted conception, and she contextualized the 'enterprising up' of conception (1997: 78) in the 1980s in relation to Thatcherite political initiatives aiming to enhance entrepreneurial activity and consumer choice. Franklin also demonstrated the ways in which notions of progress linked individual and public discourses on assisted conception, with the hope of an individual 'miracle baby' inextricably bound up with hope and faith in scientific progress. As her work illustrated, kinship links together 'the enclosed, private world of the family, and the outside world of the state's legislative apparatus and the project of nation making' (Carsten, 2004: 6).

Although the historic concerns of the field of kinship studies – kinship terminologies, rules of descent, marriage and post-marital residence – have lost their privileged place (Peletz, 1995), as the work of Franklin and others illustrates, the opening up of the field has enabled the study of kinship to extend to a diverse array of interrelated phenomena, 'from the gene to the body, the species, the family, the nation, the globe, and beyond' (Franklin and McKinnon, 2000: 279). Kinship, irrevocably dismantled as a thing-in-itself, is today broadly conceived as the study of relatedness – the ways in which people create similarity or difference between themselves and others (Carsten, 2004: 82). Anthropologists and other social scientists no longer confine their efforts to understanding the 'social' aspects of kinship, setting aside the 'biological' as pre-given, natural, and falling outside of their expertise (cf. Carsten, 2004: 6). If, as Michael Peletz (1995: 366) argues, 'developments in the new reproductive technologies make "nature" and biology more relevant to our analytic thinking about kinship than they have been since Morgan', interest now centres on the way in which the biological and social are actively produced through the conceptualization and enactment of kinship (Edwards and Salazar, 2009). These approaches are critical in a period where notions of genetic inheritance have become increasingly central to biomedical conceptions of disease.

The 'geneticization' of biomedicine: anthropological and sociological perspectives

Over the past few decades, there has been an explosion of research into genetics. The rise of what has been termed the 'new genetics' has witnessed an intense preoccupation with the possibilities of genetic technologies to prolong life, alleviate disease and obtain greater control over personal attributes such as intelligence, aggression, shyness and so on (Finkler et al., 2003). Its most ambitious manifestation to date is arguably the Human Genome Project – an international scientific research project that aims to map the human genome. The pre-eminence of the genome has led numerous observers to highlight the growing 'geneticization' of identity and to suggest that human subjects have become reduced to mere expressions of their genes (see Rose, 2007 for further discussion).

A superficial reading of the effects of these technologies might suggest that they have served to reaffirm the validity of older assumptions about the biogenetic basis of identity and relatedness – that the 'biology box' and the 'social box' can be disentangled after all (cf. Edwards, 2009: 4). There is little doubt that genetic technologies, such as the new reproductive technologies, have profound implications for the experience of kinship (see Finkler, 2000; Finkler et al., 2003; Featherstone et al., 2006; Gibbon and Novas, 2007; Edwards and Salazar, 2009). However, while genetic technologies may serve to strengthen the conventional categories of reproduction and biological relatedness (Featherstone et al., 2006), biology is no longer understood to constitute destiny, but something that can be intervened into, manipulated and transformed.[12]

For example, Carlos Novas and Nikolas Rose (2000: 487) argue that re-cataloguing illness along a genetic axis does not necessarily generate fatalism; instead, mutated forms of personhood or 'somatic individuality' arise, whereby new relations are established between body and self, 'creating an obligation to act in the present in relation to the potential futures that now come into view'.[13] Moreover, instead of leading to a focus on the individual as an isolate, individuals are subjectified through their location within networks of relatedness and obligation (Rose, 2007: 111). After all, an individual's discovery that she is 'at risk' of a specific genetic disorder has wider consequences – not just for herself but for her relatives (Featherstone et al., 2006).

As Paul Rabinow (1996) prophetically argued, the new genetics has led to the emergence of 'biosociality', a term he used to describe new forms of collectivization organized in the context of growing knowledge about genetic diseases and risks, which has seen people asserting the commonality of a shared genetic status and the new 'truths' it inscribes. These new biosocial identities, he insisted, would not straightforwardly supersede older forms of cultural classification such as race, gender and age, but would instead colonize and intersect with them in all sorts of complex (and often insidious) ways. However, as Rabinow made clear in his emphasis on the term 'biosociality', the forces he was describing were not straightforwardly sociobiological, with culture constructed on the basis of a metaphor of nature. Instead, 'Nature will be known and remade through technique and will finally become artificial, just as culture becomes natural' (Rabinow, 1996: 241–242).

Taking up Rabinow's ideas, Rayna Rapp and colleagues (2001) have observed that biosociality entails the construction of an imagined kindred, with those who 'share' a gene or chromosome for a risk or disorder felt to be related – although they illustrate that how such genetic relatedness is actually constituted is widely variable. Fundamentally entailed in biosocial formations are also *actual* kindreds. As Ian Hacking (2006: 81) asks, 'what are families or extended kinship structures if not biosocial groups?' Today, medicine increasingly identifies families genetically 'at risk' for various disorders and a 'heavy panoply of pastoral keepers… help them experience, share, intervene in, and "understand" their fate' (Rabinow, 1996: 244), primarily through the auspices of genetic counselling clinics.

Genetic counselling and notions of relatedness

Genetic counselling is the term used to describe the process whereby people at risk of an inherited disorder are advised of the probability of developing or transmitting it, and the options they have for managing these risks (Stern, 2012). Although genetic counselling is available for people at risk of a number of different types of heritable diseases, clinics are concentrated in cancer centres, along with prenatal and paediatric clinics (Stern, 2012). The isolation of the so-called 'breast cancer' genes ($BRCA_1$ and $BRCA_2$) in the 1990s served to dramatically increase the profile of genetic counselling and screening. Although these genes are thought to be responsible for only a very small proportion of breast cancers (5–10 per cent), genetic assessment for breast cancer and other types of malignancies seen to have a strong heritable component (for example, colon cancer) has become available in a number of specialist clinics (Finkler, 2000; Gibbon, 2007).

As several commentators have observed, central to these clinical encounters is the mapping of the counselee's family history (Finkler, 2000; Finkler et al., 2003; Svendsen, 2006; Gibbon, 2007). This history is condensed in the form of a kinship diagram that comprises the focus of the encounter. In much the same vein as the early generation of anthropologists – and using figures and notations that look virtually identical – the counsellor constructs a family tree (see Figure 5.2). Although this tree aims to 'get at' the genetic truths of cancer inheritance rather than the social rules of descent that so preoccupied early anthropologists, it forms a similarly fetishized object.[14] As Mette Nordahl Svendsen (2006) highlights in her work on cancer genetic counselling in Denmark, such diagrams create an image of the gene as an active agent, with persons objectified as nodes in a web of biological relationships and as a phase the gene enters on its route through time.

The story invoked in counselling sessions is one of the force and sway of genetic ties in the inexorable movement of cancer-causing genes through generations via the reproductive acts that carry them forward (Svendsen, 2006). As Sahra Gibbon (2007) similarly observes in her work at breast cancer genetic counselling clinics in England, the authority and power of such statements derives in part from a particular origin story about genes, identity and reproduction, one that replicates a perceived notion of kinship predicated on biogenetic connections. On the basis of this geneticized visual representation of family history, a risk estimate is provided – both for persons in the counselling session and their family members (Gibbon, 2007: 51). The family tree thus governs the type of intervention offered to patients (Gibbon, 2007: 52).[15]

However, although the family tree provides a framework for conceptualizing the journey of the gene through time, creating a future of continuous illness, it simultaneously evokes the possibility of intervention to 'control the forces of the

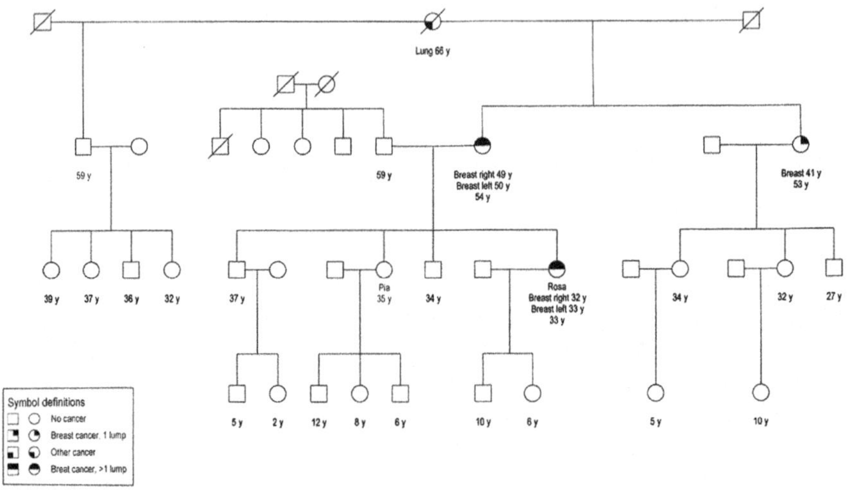

FIGURE 5.2 Extract of a family tree produced by a genetic counsellor for sisters 'Rosa' and 'Pia' (Source: cancer genetic counselling clinic in Denmark, reproduced with permission from Svendsen, 2006).

gene and to secure a future of survival' (Svendsen, 2006: 147). For example, women carrying mutations in the BRCA genes are now conceptualized as 'previvors': '*sur-vivors* of a *pre*disposition to cancer' (FORCE, 2011) and are offered risk-reduction drugs like tamoxifen, along with more invasive options such as prophylactic mastectomies (see Gibbon, 2007; Fosket, 2010).[16]

The actress Angelina Jolie's decision to undergo the operation following her diagnosis as a $BRCA_1$ carrier is a case in point. In describing her experience in a *New York Times* editorial, she stated: 'Once I knew that this was my reality, I decided to be proactive and to minimize the risk as much as I could' (Jolie, 2013). As Novas and Rose's (2000) description of 'somatic individuality' suggests, evident in Jolie's account is the moral imperative that such screening creates to 'do something'. In her words: 'Life comes with many challenges. The ones that should not scare us are the ones we can take on and take control of' (Jolie, 2013). Also evoked in Jolie's account is a sense of the power of biogenetic ties and the triumph of medicine over them. The article begins with her mother's story – 'my mother fought cancer for almost a decade and died at 56' – and emphasizes that this story will not be the one Jolie's own children tell: 'I can tell my children that they don't need to fear they will lose me to breast cancer.' Here, the reader is presented with an account of biology, interrupted.[17]

As accounts by social scientists make clear, while genetic counselling ostensibly 'fixes' biological ties, it also serves to reconfigure kinship knowledge in complex ways (Finkler, 2000; Svendsen, 2006). Svendsen (2006) describes the processes through which genetic counselling sessions simultaneously denaturalize and reinscribe notions of biological relatedness. According to Svendsen, this literalization of biological kinship in the course of the counselling session exposes such relations as contingent, as counselees come to see the disjunctures between those blood relatives they have social relationships with versus those they don't (and conversely their sense of relatedness to those affinal kin erased on the family tree). In other words, it reveals that experiences of kinship and relatedness are based on factors *other than* biology (see also Finkler, 2000, for similar illustrations). However, relationships are simultaneously rebiologized as social contact with biological relatives is constructed as being both necessary and natural.[18] As Svendsen notes, the family tree serves to construct a form of biosociality, as shared genetic status becomes the basis of a sense of connection and family members are mobilized around the biological issue of pursuing knowledge about genetic risks. In her words: 'The production of genetic knowledge in counselling depends on treating biological ties as something that make certain kinds of social relationships possible' (Svendsen, 2006: 148).

The medicalization of kinship that genetic counselling facilitates comes across strongly in Kaja Finkler's (2000) US research with women with breast cancer and a family history of the disease. For example, she documents the case of 'Eve', a 59-year-old woman whose mother died of breast cancer at the age of 34, who experienced herself as 'sitting on a time bomb' because of her family history of cancer. Eve highlighted the ways in which she had become closer to her cousins: 'Knowing that they share the same genes provides the occasion for discussion... The fact that they have the same genes has created a close bond' (Finkler, 2000: 63–64). The medicalization of kinship ties became particularly evident in the case of adoptees Finkler interviewed. For example, 'Monica', a 40-year-old woman, sought out her birth parents in large part because of a desire to know more about her family's medical history. In Monica's words, 'I've had a lot of medical problems and my little boy has asthma and I have asthma and I've had two lumps removed from my breast, so I was concerned if there was cancer in the family and different things' (Finkler, 2000: 144). Her discovery of a history of heart disease and cancer in her birth family served to create a link to her birth kin and a sense of vigilance around the need to undergo regular monitoring for both conditions.

However, Finkler's work also illustrates the ways in which women resisted the medicalization of kinship. 'Karen', a 39-year-old woman whose mother and grandmother had died of breast cancer, referred to her mother, father, brother, and mother and father's siblings as her 'relatives', but she did not regard her cousins as 'family', in clear contrast to her genetic counsellor. In fact, apparent in many women's accounts was the ways they both invoked and rejected the biological basis of kinship, depending on the specific context. As Carles Salazar (2009) observes, for genetic knowledge to be relevant in a particular kinship system, genes must have cultural value; in other words, they must be meaningful in terms of the kinship system and not merely 'true' in biological terms. In his words, 'the existence of these biological ties, a truth knowledge, does not necessarily mean that they have to be socially significant in any way' (Salazar, 2009: 192). Instead, he argues that it is the kinship system itself – as a tool of translation between nature and culture – that has played a crucial role in the emergence of the symbolic power of genes. In the words of Franklin and McKinnon, kinship moves 'back and forth between what counts as natural/given and cultural/created. In the process, kinship becomes the site for producing what will count as the *difference* between nature and culture' (2001: 61, emphasis in original).

Conclusion

Anthropologists have always been aware that kinship is something more than an expression of blood ties, and this recognition explains much of the discipline's long-standing preoccupation with the topic. Although early anthropological theories assumed the biogenetic basis of kinship, over time it became increasingly difficult to sustain a distinction between the 'natural' facts of kinship and their 'cultural' elaboration. As we have seen elsewhere (see especially Chapter 3), anthropologists engaged with ethnographic worlds that could not be fully contained by their theories and interpretations.

Although attempts to rethink kinship were a feature of kinship studies throughout the twentieth century, it was the emergence of new reproductive technologies – and anthropological and sociological efforts to grapple with them – that were instrumental in the transformation of the field. These works revealed that kinship was not a thing-in-itself that could be studied in isolation from other aspects of society. Moreover, rather than constituting an insoluble building block out of which kinship was forged, nature was not the fixed and stable category priorly assumed.

As such studies illustrate, in much the same way that 'culture' has been utilized as a way of identifying, naming and marking out difference (see Chapter 1), 'kinship' is similarly a means of producing notions of difference and sameness – albeit in this case between 'culture' and 'nature'. In other words, kinship is a key site 'in which distinctions between nature and culture, what is given and what is acquired, what is fixed and what is changeable, are produced' (Edwards, 2009: 9). Although the rise of the new reproductive technologies and the new genetics may have blurred the boundaries between what is attributable to nature and what is attributable to culture, these concepts still form central organizing principles in our understanding of such technologies – and the social, political and ethical dilemmas they raise. Thus, despite the waxing and waning status of the concept of kinship over the past century, the fact that it takes on the nature–culture tension is likely to ensure its durability well into the future.

Notes

1 For example, see E.E. Evans-Pritchard's (1940: 12–13) discussion of 'Neurosis'; and Napoleon Chagnon (1997 [1968]: 19–21) and Claude Lévi-Strauss's (1992: 279) accounts of the lengths they went to to elicit kinship names and genealogies among the Yąnomamö and Nambikwara respectively.

2 Nor do I cross into distinctly sociological studies of kinship with an emphasis on the family (as an institution), social networks, community and fragmentation (see Young and Willmott, 1957; Morgan, 1996; Smart and Neale, 1999).
3 The influence of Morgan's work was felt well beyond the realm of anthropology and was a key inspiration for Friedrich Engels' 1884 book *Origins of the Family, Private Property and the State in Light of Researches of Lewis H. Morgan*, which itself was instrumental in the development of Marxist theories of production (see Chapter 4 for further details).
4 Radcliffe-Brown (1929: 50) highlighted various 'misconceptions' in Rivers' work on Ambrym kinship, and the ways his assumptions about kinship formations 'unconsciously' influenced his inquiries.
5 A unilineal descent group is one in which descent is traced through either the female (matrilineal descent) or male line (patrilineal descent).
6 See Chapter 6 for further explications of Lévi-Strauss's work on exchange.
7 See especially Rosaldo and Lamphere (1974) and MacCormack and Strathern (1980).
8 However, the intersections are clearly complicated. For example, contributors to *Nature, Culture and Gender* (MacCormack and Strathern, 1980) and *Woman, Culture and Society* (Rosaldo and Lamphere, 1974) were clearly influenced by Schneider's earlier work on kinship.
9 As Carsten (2004) observes, although the tendency to distinguish between attributes that are seen as innate and those that are seen as acquired may be universal, *what* is regarded as innate or acquired and *how* sameness and difference are construed cannot be cordoned off in advance.
10 This is the title of Marilyn Strathern's (1992a) influential book.
11 It is also evident in recent UK debates about the introduction of laws that will allow the creation of babies from the DNA of three people in order to stop genetic diseases being passed from mother to child – see the Conclusion for further discussion.
12 Katie Featherstone and her colleagues (2006) argue that although new genetic technologies and new reproductive technologies tend to be conflated by scholars writing about kinship, these technologies operate differently, with the latter weakening the perceived relationships between the biological 'facts' of conception and the social categories of kinship and the former strengthening them. However, in both cases the nature/culture dichotomy is ultimately destabilized. Moreover, as Jeanette Edwards (2009: 12) points out, juxtaposing these technologies can provoke 'analogies and connections that illuminate rather than obscure'.
13 See Chapter 7 for an illustration of these points in relation to the rise of neuroscientific approaches to addiction.
14 See Mary Bouquet (1993) on the fetishization of the family tree in anthropological studies of kinship and Mette Nordahl Svendsen (2006) and Sahra Gibbon (2007) on its parallel role in genetic counselling.
15 For example, it generally determines whether genetic testing is warranted.
16 It's worth noting that there are differences in the degree of endorsement of prophylactic mastectomies across national settings. For example, early French clinical guidelines were more stringent than their US counterpart in terms of the contexts in which it was recommended (see Eisinger et al., 1999) and substantial differences have more recently been found between France, Germany, the Netherlands and the UK in terms of physicians' attitudes towards the procedure (Den Heijer et al., 2013).
17 I could not help this allusion to *Girl, Interrupted*, the film for which Jolie won an Academy Award in 2000.
18 Although it is assumed that risk disclosure will happen within the family when one member is discovered to be at genetic risk for an inherited condition, it's worth noting that communication about genetic risk in the family is far from straightforward. A growing body of literature documents the complicated ethics of genetic testing in terms of obligations to disclose (O'Doherty, 2014) and gender, ethnic, class and cultural differences in patterns of disclosure (Shaw and Hurst, 2009).

References

Bouquet, M. (1993) *Reclaiming English Kinship: Portuguese Refractions of British Kinship Theory*. Manchester: Manchester University Press.

Carsten, J. (2004) *After Kinship*. Cambridge: Cambridge University Press.

Chagnon, N. (1997 [1968]) *Yąnomamö*. Belmont, CA: Wadsworth.

Collier, J.F. and Yanagisako, S.J. (eds.) (1987) *Gender and Kinship: Essays Toward a Unified Analysis*. Stanford, CA: Stanford University Press.

Den Heijer, M., van Asperen, C.J., Harris, H., Nippert, I., Schmidtke, J., Bouhnik, A.D., Julian-Reynier, C., Evans, D.G. and Tibben, A. (2013) International variation in physicians' attitudes towards prophylactic mastectomy – comparison between France, Germany, the Netherlands and the United Kingdom. *European Journal of Cancer*, 49(13): 2798–2805.

Dumont, L. (2006 [1971]) *Introduction to Two Theories of Social Anthropology: Descent Groups and Marriage Alliance*. Edited and translated by R. Parkin. New York: Berghahn Books.

Edwards, J. (2009) Introduction: the matter in kinship. In J. Edwards and C. Salazar (eds.), *European Kinship in the Age of Biotechnology*. New York: Berghahn Books, 1–18.

Edwards, J. and Salazar, C. (eds.) (2009) *European Kinship in the Age of Biotechnology*. New York: Berghahn Books.

Eisinger, F., Geller, G., Burke, W. and Holtzman, N.A. (1999) Cultural basis for differences between US and French clinical recommendations for women at increased risk of breast and ovarian cancer. *The Lancet*, 353: 919–920.

Engels, F. (1972 [1884]) *Origins of the Family, Private Property and the State in Light of Researches of Lewis H. Morgan*. Atlanta, GA: Pathfinder Press.

Evans-Pritchard, E.E. (1940) *The Nuer: A Description of the Modes of Livelihood and Political Institutions of a Nilotic People*. New York: Oxford University Press.

Featherstone, K., Atkinson, P., Bharadwaj, A. and Clarke, A. (2006) *Risky Relations: Family, Kinship and the New Genetics*. Oxford: Berg.

Finkler, K. (2000) *Experiencing the New Genetics: Family and Kinship on the Medical Frontier*. Philadelphia, PA: University of Pennsylvania Press.

Finkler, K., Skrzynia, C. and Evans, J.P. (2003) The new genetics and its consequences for family, kinship, medicine and medical genetics. *Social Science and Medicine*, 57: 403–412.

FORCE (2011) Cancer previvors, in *FORCE: Facing Our Risk of Cancer Empowered*, www.facingourrisk.org/info_research/previvors-survivors/cancer-previvors/index.php.

Fosket, J.R. (2010) Breast cancer risk as disease. In A.E. Clarke, L. Mamo, J.R. Fosket, J.R. Fishman and J. Shim (eds.), *Biomedicalization: Technoscience, Health and Illness in the US*. Durham: Duke University Press, 331–352.

Fox, R. (1967) *Kinship and Marriage*. Harmondsworth: Penguin Books.

Franklin, S. (1997) *Embodied Progress: a Cultural Account of Assisted Conception*. London: Routledge.

Franklin, S. and McKinnon, S. (2000) New directions in kinship study: a core concept revisited. *Current Anthropology*, 41(2): 275–279.

Franklin, S. and McKinnon, S. (eds.) (2001) *Relative Values: Reconfiguring Kinship Studies*. Durham, NC: Duke University Press.

Gibbon, S. (2007) *Breast Cancer Genes and the Gendering of Knowledge*. London: Palgrave Macmillan.

Gibbon, S. and Novas, C. (eds.) (2007) *Biosocialities, Genetics and the Social Sciences: Making Biologies and Identities*. London: Routledge.

Hacking, I. (2006) Genetics, biosocial groups and the future of identity. *Daedalus*, Fall: 81–95.

Holy, L. (1996) *Anthropological Perspectives on Kinship*. London: Pluto Press.

Jolie, A. (2013) My medical choice. *New York Times*, May 14: A25.

Leach, E.R. (1961) *Rethinking Anthropology*. London: Athlone Press.

Lévi-Strauss, C. (1969) *The Elementary Structures of Kinship*. Boston, MA: Beacon Press.

Lévi-Strauss, C. (1992) *Tristes Tropiques*. Translated by J. Weightman and D. Weightman. New York: Penguin Books.

MacCormack, C. and Strathern, M. (1980) *Nature, Culture and Gender*. Cambridge: Cambridge University Press.

Malinowski, B. (1929) *The Sexual Life of Savages: An Ethnographic Account of Courtship, Marriage and Family Life Among the Natives of the Trobriand Highlands, British New Guinea*. Boston, MA: Beacon Press.

Malinowski, B. (1930) Kinship. *Man*, 30: 19–29.

Morgan, D. (1996) *Family Connections: An Introduction to Family Studies*. Cambridge: Polity Press.

Morgan, L.H. (1985 [1877]) *Ancient Society: Researches in the Lines of Human Progress From Savagery Through Barbarism to Civilization*. Tucson, AZ: University of Arizona Press.

Needham, R. (ed.) (1971) *Rethinking Kinship and Marriage*. London: Tavistock.

Novas, C. and Rose, N. (2000) Genetic risk and the birth of the somatic individual. *Economy and Society*, 29(4): 485–513.

O'Doherty, K. (2014) Genetic counselling, overview. *Encyclopedia of Critical Psychology*, 774–779.

Parkin, R. (2006) Editor's introduction. In L. Dumont, *Introduction to Two Theories of Social Anthropology: Descent Groups and Marriage Alliance*. New York: Berghahn Books, vii–xxx.

Peletz, M. (1995) Kinship studies in late twentieth century anthropology. *Annual Review of Anthropology*, 24: 343–372.

Rabinow, P. (1996) *Essays on the Anthropology of Reason*. Princeton, NJ: Princeton University Press.

Radcliffe-Brown, A.R. (1929) A further note on Ambrym. *Man*, 29: 50–53.

Radcliffe-Brown, A.R. (1950) Introduction. In A.R. Radcliffe-Brown and D. Forde (eds.), *African Systems of Kinship and Marriage*. London: Oxford University Press, 1–85.

Rapp, R., Heath, D. and Taussig, K-S. (2001) Geneaological dis-ease: where hereditary abnormality, biomedical explanation, and family responsibility meet. In S. Franklin and S. McKinnon (eds.), *Relative Values: Reconfiguring Kinship Studies*. Durham, NC: Duke University Press, 384–411.

Rivers, W.H.R. (1900) A genealogical method of collecting social and vital statistics. *Journal of the Anthropological Institute of Great Britain and Ireland*, 30: 74–82.

Rivers, W.H.R. (1910) The genealogical method of anthropological inquiry. *Sociological Review*, 3: 1–12.

Rosaldo, R.Z. and Lamphere, L. (1974) *Woman, Culture and Society*. Stanford, CA: Stanford University Press.

Rose, N. (2007) *The Politics of Life Itself*. Princeton, NJ: Princeton University Press.

Salazar, C. (2009) Are genes good to think with? In J. Edwards and C. Salazar (eds.), *European Kinship in the Age of Biotechnology*. New York: Berghahn Books, 179–196.

Schneider, D.M. (1980 [1968]) *American Kinship: A Cultural Account*, 2nd edn. Chicago: University of Chicago Press.

Schneider, D.M. (1984) *A Critique of the Study of Kinship*. Ann Arbor, MI: University of Michigan Press.

Shaw, A. and Hurst, J.A. (2009) 'I don't see any point in telling them': attitudes to sharing genetic information in the family and carrier testing of relatives among British Pakistani adults referred to a genetics clinic. *Ethnicity and Health*, 14(2): 205–224.

Smart, C. and Neale, B. (1999) *Family Fragments*. Cambridge: Polity Press.

Stern, A.M. (2012) *Telling Genes: the Story of Genetic Counseling in America*. Baltimore, MD: Johns Hopkins University Press.

Strathern, M. (1992a) *After Nature: English Kinship in the Late Twentieth Century*. Cambridge: Cambridge University Press.

Strathern, M. (1992b) *Reproducing the Future: Essays on Anthropology, Kinship and the New Reproductive Technologies*. Manchester: Manchester University Press.

Svendsen, M.N. (2006) The social life of genetic knowledge: a case-study of choices and dilemmas in cancer genetic counselling in Denmark. *Medical Anthropology*, 25(2): 139–170.

Trautman, T. (1987) *Lewis Henry Morgan and the Invention of Kinship*. Berkeley: University of California Press.

Young, M. and Willmott, P. (1957) *Family and Kinship in East London*. London: Routledge.

6

EXCHANGE

Ciara Kierans

> What power resides in the object given that causes its recipient to pay it back?
>
> Marcel Mauss, *The Gift*

Introduction

In an article on the subject of doing harm in the context of *living* organ donation published in the *Journal of Medical Ethics*, Carl Elliot (1995) draws attention to Graham Greene's (1985) novella, *The Tenth Man*. Greene's novel tells the story of a French lawyer, Louis Chavel, jailed during World War II by the Nazis. The book begins one week after his imprisonment. The 29 other men sharing the prison camp are drawn from various walks of life, and include engine drivers, barbers, greengrocers, tobacconists and clerks, as well as a mayor. From the outset, Chavel struggles with his imprisonment and the proximity it forces with men of lower social status. He sees the majority of his cellmates as 'natural prisoners, who would have found themselves prisoners in any case sooner or later… – while he himself was a prisoner by mistake' (Greene, 1985: 34).

Following news that the Resistance have murdered some townspeople, a prison guard informs the assembled prisoners that three men will be shot. The guard continues: 'We are quite indifferent as to which three. You can choose for yourselves. The funeral rites will begin at seven tomorrow morning' (Greene, 1985: 40). After some discussion among the prisoners about how to choose the unlucky three, the mayor suggests that they draw lots – 'it is the only fair thing' (1985: 40). The lots are drawn, and Chavel is among the three marked for death. Unlike the other two men, Voisin and Lenôtre, who stoically accept the outcome, Chavel panics. Hysterical, he offers 100,000 francs to anyone who will take the marker. When this proclamation solicits no takers, he offers 'everything I've got… money, land, everything'

(1985: 47). To the astonishment of all, Janvier, a sickly young clerk, accepts on the condition that Chavel draws up a will for him leaving everything to his mother and sister. Voisin bitterly notes, 'we can't buy *our* lives… It's not fair' (1985: 49, emphasis in original), a feeling clearly shared by the majority of prisoners. Janvier, Voisin and Lenôtre are shot the next morning and Chavel realizes that while he has survived, he is 'one of them now, a man without money or position' (1985: 59).

A series of events lead Chavel to his old estate where Janvier's mother and sister, Thérèse, are now ensconced. Under an assumed name, he takes a temporary position with the family as an odd-job man. Although Janvier's mother believes her son to still be alive, Thérèse, who knows the truth of her brother's death, is far from grateful at Janvier's actions on his family's behalf. There, Chavel is forced to recognize the far-reaching implications of his actions, on not just Janvier himself but his family.

As Elliot's analysis makes clear, the story is not simply about an exchange between two men: an autonomous act, individually entered into. The exchange in the story is one that establishes the grounds of a gift that will ostensibly give Janvier's mother and sister a much better life. The entangled acts of requesting and giving are, at once, intensely complex personal, social, political and moral phenomena that always have consequences far beyond the immediacy of the initial exchange. For Elliot, the question is, given this, whether we ought to encourage individuals to undergo harm for the good of another and, in turn, whether we ought to encourage individuals to take advantage of another's sacrifice.

The complex social arrangements that various forms of exchange give rise to constitute important concerns for the social sciences today, concerns that have their foundations in earlier anthropological work.[1] For anthropologists, exchange relationships are neither discrete nor dyadic, but are woven into and so are deeply reflective of the social fabric out of which they are made. Instances of gift-giving fulfil complex demands and expectations that structure and give form to the everyday lives of families, communities and societies, as the ethnographic record richly attests. Fundamental are the profound social relations that are established and sustained through its practice (Laidlaw, 2000). Gift exchange is both a pragmatic and symbolic exercise, one in which we see the forces of culture clearly at play (see Chapter 1).

This chapter focuses on the act of giving within the context of biotechnological practices. It is concerned with the pivotal role of the body and its parts as things increasingly to be exchanged. To illustrate, I focus on the role of blood, organs and whole bodies as phenomena bound up with complex modes of transfer. Gift-giving, as the central trope and point of departure, is one firmly fastened to the academic and popular imagination. I trace its emergence and discuss its significance, starting with the seminal work of Marcel Mauss in his classic essay, *The Gift*.

The gift: social bonds – material and symbolic values

Mauss, the nephew of the French sociologist Émile Durkheim, published *The Gift* in 1925. Its focus was the character of reciprocal exchange within what he referred to as 'primitive' or 'archaic' societies such as the Tlingit, Haida and Kwakiutl (Pacific Northwest) and the Maori (New Zealand), societies, which anthropologists have also described as non-market or kin-ordered (Wolf, 1982). In such contexts, gift-giving constituted a practice in which symbolism and materiality were interdependent, as the exchange of things between people was organized and ritualized by social norms and customs. Mauss showed that gifts, as the primary mode of the exchange, are neither voluntary nor disinterested but, in fact, obligatory and interested. They are fundamentally characterized by tripartite social relations: the requirement to give, to receive and, in turn, to reciprocate. Bound to the exchange is the symbolic and transcendent character of giving. As gifts are understood to be ultimately part of or tied to the giver, the giver inevitably gives part of themselves: their spirit – their life force or '*hau*' in Maori terms. Gift-giving embodies the specificity of social relations in a particular place, at a particular time. It ensures that people within a society are fully wedded to the things they produce and exchange (Taussig, 1980).[2] Solidarities are, therefore, implicit in the process, and the failure to engage or reciprocate the exchange is tantamount to a declaration of war – a refusal of friendship and intercourse (Johansen, 1967).

While Mauss began the work of systematizing the analysis of gift-giving as a cultural practice, he took his lead from Bronisław Malinowski's prior research on the Kula Ring, a system of reciprocal exchange among the Trobriand Islanders. In that research Malinowski documented how island traders travelled by canoe across hundreds of miles of water between archipelagos to exchange bracelets (*mwali*) and necklaces (*soulava*), each moving in opposite directions. These goods remained temporarily with the receiver before they were exchanged again. Writing in *Argonauts of the Western Pacific* (1922), Malinowski rhetorically asked why men would risk life and limb to travel across huge expanses of dangerous ocean to give away what appear to be worthless trinkets. His analysis proceeded to show these exchanges as essentially non-altruistic, bound up with the purpose of enhancing status and prestige. Giving was politically motivated, with the giver expected to make a return of equal or greater value. Malinowski's message was clear: there could be no giving without reciprocity. Where Malinowski put emphasis on practices of exchange undertaken by individuals as individuals, Mauss noted that exchange was also crucial in cementing links and settling differences of rank and worth among those who positioned themselves as representatives of social groupings or collectives. In such contexts, gift systems were 'total prestations', the outcome of reciprocal obligations through which the gift itself came to embody the identity or 'spirit' of its 'corporate' giver – indeed, where the repeat cycle of gift and return gift came to define the whole social order.

What motivates such reciprocal exchanges has provoked considerable debate, particularly among economic and political anthropologists. Malinowski and Mauss, despite their differences, both shared the view that gift exchange was not a discrete practice but one that served a wide range of functions – in terms of renewing kinship bonds, religious connections, political ties and economic relationships – on the basis of which the local character of the practice takes its particular forms (Sahlins, 1972; Parry, 1986).

Expanding on this insight, Marshall Sahlins (1972) characterized Mauss's notion of the gift as reflecting a *generalized* mode of reciprocity, commonly understood at the level of the household – a system of exchange where there is an implicit expectation that a return will be made, but with no attempt to keep track of the value or the debt. He contrasted this with *balanced or symmetrical reciprocity* – where the value and timing of the return is anticipated – and *negative reciprocity* – where the capacity to profit from the exchange shapes the relations of exchange. For Sahlins, the more integrated and close-knit the society is, the more likely it is to rely on forms of gift exchange. He thus stressed the differing social and political contexts – and consequences – each model entailed.

The intrinsically political character of gift-giving is illustrated in two well-known ethnographic examples: the Moka and the Potlatch. The Moka is a form of exchange found in Papua New Guinea, made famous through the work of Marshall Sahlins (1963) and Andrew Strathern's ethnographic film *Ongka's Big Moka* (1974). Contrasted with the processes and practices of formal political states, Sahlins describes how power and prestige manifest through the display of 'Big Man' politics, itself underpinned by the reciprocal gifting of pigs. The essence of the Moka is not in the exchange itself but the increment or extra value that one is expected to provide through the act of reciprocation.

A similar emphasis on power and prestige is evident in the 'Potlatch': a gift-giving feast found most notably among the peoples of the Pacific Northwest coast (Boas, 1888; Godelier, 1999). Organized and held to mark significant ceremonies such as births, deaths, weddings or the formation of alliances, the Potlatch is, at once, a mode of distribution of goods and a strategy for the maintenance of power and stability. Hosted only by those of rank and status, Potlatches incurred the obligation to give away (or destroy) all worldly goods as a marker of office and power. If a guest did not, in turn, reciprocate by hosting bigger feasts, giving away more goods, they (and their people) stood to lose 'face' and power. Mauss (1967: 4) referred to the Potlatch as 'essentially usurious and extravagant… above all a struggle among nobles to determine their position in the hierarchy to the ultimate benefit'.

Potlatching in North America was outlawed towards the end of the nineteenth century, as the social forms it was grounded in collided with the principles of surplus accumulation and the commodity form (Boas, 1888; Cole and Chaikin, 1990). It was, when seen from the perspective of the new colonial authorities, thought of as being a shamelessly wasteful and unproductive exercise, contrary to those *civilized* values embedded in mechanisms of market exchange (see Nash, 1979; Taussig, 1980 for critiques on the implications of new commodity forms on non-market societies). As a consequence of their focus on situations such as these, where systems of exchange clash, some anthropologists have tended to treat gift and commodity forms in a polarized fashion (for discussion see Gregory, 1982). However, others have resisted the tendency to see any value in juxtapositions, and have focused instead on their interpenetrations (Appadurai, 1986; Strathern, 1988; Thomas, 1991) – a concern taken up in later sections. The idea, however, that reciprocal exchange is pervasive across cultures and has an enduring role within social interaction has persuaded some of its universal character. Claude Lévi-Strauss (1969 [1949]) claimed three domains of reciprocal exchange underpinning *all* human relationships: the exchange of words (language), the exchange of women (kinship) and that of things (economics). Others, by contrast, have challenged the very existence of a thing call called a 'gift economy', insisting, as Malinowski and Mauss might have, that systems of exchange only acquire their particular character (political, religious, kinship) within the context of the systems and practices of which they are a part (Parry, 1986; Godelier, 1999; Weiner, 1992; Graeber, 2001).

Despite these disputes, anthropologists, alongside many others within the social sciences, continue to find the gift indispensable. It is a concept continually put to work, particularly in the domain of medicine and healthcare, where an increasing range of goods and services are mobilized for exchange purposes. In the next section, we follow some of these goods through another seminal study – Richard Titmuss's (1970) classic *The Gift Relationship*. While not an anthropological study per se, it was certainly influenced by anthropological perspectives and, in turn, has generated new problems and questions for the discipline. Titmuss's project, moreover, concerns a substance explored in the context of kinship in Chapter 5 – that of blood and its unique capacity to reveal social and cultural formations and mobilize diverse and complex transactional forms.[3] Blood has, in addition, immense methodological value for social scientists, in that it functions as a vector between domains that in other contexts are kept apart. As these include the domains of family, ritual and religion, medicine and the market (Carsten, 2011), they enable access to the multi-sited character of medicalized things, processes and practices (Appadurai, 1986; Marcus, 1998).

Blood: transfers and transfusions

Drawing on Mauss's key insight that gifts are not predicated on the exchange of things but on the formation and maintenance of relationships, Titmuss, in response to proposals for market-based – i.e., paid – blood donation, argued the merits of gift exchange over the commodity form: of public over private healthcare and the welfare state over the market. Focusing on the differences between the organization of blood services in the US and UK, he observed that in the latter system the exchange of blood was supported by the National Blood Service, an organization dependent on voluntary donations to blood banks across all social classes. Titmuss (1970) advocated this model as a standardized and secure system that distributed important blood supplies according to need with little wastage – all driven by an ethos of social solidarity and human empathy. By comparison, the supply of blood in the US was characterized by fragmentation and a mix of public and private forms. Voluntary organizations such as the Red Cross operated alongside for-profit community blood banks. Because the system relied on payments in cash or credit, Titmuss contended that the American blood supply was inefficient, wasteful and expensive. Moreover, reliance on the 'cash nexus', i.e., a system of payments through which individuals could command commodities within a market, contaminated not only healthcare in general but the blood system in particular. This argument has had an enduring influence on transfusion and transplantation discourses and policy literatures and is regularly drawn on as a challenge to market-driven strategies to healthcare provision.

Although Titmuss endorsed the generalized reciprocity characterizing the UK system as superior to the US model, with its commodity-based mode of exchange ('negative reciprocity' in Sahlins' framing), a third 'replacement' model of blood donation exists in many parts of the world. Characterized by a form of balanced or symmetrical reciprocity, this family-based system of donation is the norm in countries such as India and involves a family member donating blood to replace the blood withdrawn from the bank to treat an ailing relative (Copeman, 2009a, 2009b). In such systems, blood donation relies on the perceived power and force of kinship ties to ensure that blood 'withdrawals' are 'repaid' – a debt is incurred and absolved. Nevertheless, despite the existence of alternatives beyond the US market-based model, Titmuss's insistence on the superiority of voluntary, non-remunerated donation within an anonymous system of procurement has become standard orthodoxy among powerful agencies such as the World Health Organization and the Red Cross. There is thus considerable pressure on countries with replacement systems in place to implement this model, with its underlying prioritization of notions of altruism and disinterestedness.

While Titmuss's work has been enormously influential, his analysis is not without limitations. Reflecting the scientific orthodoxies of his time, Titmuss could not have anticipated the wider technological advances that now shape the uses to which blood, as a donated gift, is put (Waldby and Mitchell, 2006) – uses that threaten the arguments he presented. Before the twentieth century, blood was assumed to be a uniform, discrete substance shared by all humans. However, in the early twentieth century, this view was shown to be false when Karl Landsteiner discovered the significance of blood types. Over the following decades, this discovery prompted the search for greater blood-borne differences across populations and a growing racialization of blood types. Arthur Mourant, who pioneered the classification and mapping of blood groups across populations in the 1950s, made full use of anthropological investigations as opportunities for the collection of blood samples for research and indexing purposes. Anthropological data was drawn on as the standard form for classifying populations – in recognized racial and ethnic terms – and genetic information was calibrated to reflect its categorizations, serving to turn established tribal and ethnic groups into biologically/genetically *readable* entities. This has had profound implications not only for the exchange and movement of blood between bodies, but practically too – most significantly in the ways in which blood is collected, stored, labelled and administered.

The segregation of blood products by race has impacted widely on who may give to whom, a subject that has, over the latter part of the twentieth century, been hotly contested socially, culturally and politically (for discussion on the exchange of organs in the context of race, see Chapter 1). The American Red Cross, for example, maintained racial tags on blood until 1950, while controversies over blood exchanges gave rise to high-profile civil rights cases in the USA during the 1960s and 1970s (Lederer, 2008). More recently, concerns (often initially flagged by anthropologists) have been raised about the ways in which the classificatory apparatuses of blood substances are mobilized to mark out the emergence of 'ethnic' diseases in the context of the 'new genetics' (Gordon, 2002; Duster, 2005; Fullwiley, 2008; Fausto-Sterling, 2008; Avera, 2009; Kierans and Cooper, 2011).

The problematic status and stability of blood as a substance and its role as an identity marker does not surface in *The Gift Relationship*. Instead, the fact that blood does not allow for straightforward or discrete exchanges between parties has led many to challenge the sense in which it can be accorded the status of a gift, something taken up by Catherine Waldby and Robert Mitchell (2006) in *Tissue Economies*. Waldby and Mitchell contend that the reliance on the inherent moral and distributive qualities of gift systems is no longer adequate in the context of blood exchange. Since the mid-1970s, blood has rarely been transfused whole but is now fractioned into a number of components – plasma, red cells, white cells and platelets – to be provided to multiple recipients. Because of this, blood 'is thus transformed from an act of direct civic responsibility between fellow citizens into a complex network of donor-recipient relations heavily mediated by biotechnical processes and an institutional complex of tissue banks, pharmaceutical and research companies and clinics' (Waldby and Mitchell, 2006: 22). Thus, what may begin as a gift ends up as a commodity, sourced, processed and sold by transnational pharmacology companies. The international circulation of blood products and Factor VIII[4] contrasts with whole blood whose limited lifespan restricted it to transfers within national settings, but upon which Titmuss based his analysis. Moreover, blood can be cloned and 'immortalized' by the production of cell lines or gene sequences, processes that extend life into new patentable products. It is by virtue of biotechnical developments such as these that new forms of surplus come to be increasingly generated from diverse forms of life (Cooper, 2008). In consequence, gift-commodity distinctions or juxtapositions cease to hold ground in the face of new and overlapping systems of translation, negotiation and production (Appadurai, 1986; Callon, 1998).

Biotechnical possibilities have opened up all manner of problems and questions for anthropologists about the transnational nature of blood and its modes of circulation (Anagnost, 2006; Shao, 2006). In response, anthropologists' attempts to address these problems by tracing the movement of blood have focused attention on the particular local forms blood transfer takes within increasingly globalized arrangements and, through this, have given rise to new ways of conceptualizing the relationship between risk, infection and solidarity (Shao, 2006; Shao and Scoggin, 2009). The consequences for new forms of kinship, somatic relatedness and biosociality have also been the focus of some interest (see Chapter 5), along with the changing mechanisms for shaping new constituencies of blood donors and receivers (Copeman, 2009a, 2009b). The consequences of blood transfers for identity politics, particularly those bound up with race and class (Robertson, 2002; Busby, 2004) and forms of economic citizenship (Reddy, 2007) have also been explored, along with the persistent ways in which blood donation brings to view the overlap between national commitments and religious beliefs, particularly in the context of war, conflict and violence (Simpson, 2009). Finally, social scientists have also studied the ways in which the changing technological landscape and possibilities of blood challenge the discursive and rhetorical possibilities of giving and receiving (Dalsgaard, 2007).

Organ transplantation and the metaphorical limits of the gift

Solid organ transplantation, of kidneys, hearts, lungs and so on, appears, at least superficially, to overcome one of the challenges to blood exchange in that organs have the appearance of discrete 'components': actual things to be exchanged. Considered to be one of the quintessential modern biotechnical 'advances', organ transplantation – especially of kidneys, the type of organ that will provide the focus here – has generated much interest among anthropologists, by virtue of its capacity to produce and reproduce various social, cultural and ethical concerns and controversies (Fox and Swazey, 1974; Cohen, 1999; Hogle, 1999; Scheper-Hughes, 2000; Sharp, 2001, 2006; Lock, 2001; Gordon, 2002; Crowley-Matoka, 2005; Hamdy, 2010; Kierans and Cooper, 2011). Organ transplantation raises questions about what it means to be human; the various ways in which the boundaries between life and death come to be organized; the status of body–machine hybridizations and the moral responsibilities attached to kinship and community. It also questions the role of capital and the state in supporting transplant technologies; the significance and implications of gift-giving and reciprocal exchange and the differentially situated ways in which the technologies of transplantation come to be indigenized and made to work across global settings. Continued developments in the field of transplant medicine show how tendencies towards altruism, commerce, gifting, stealing, choice and coercion overlap in profound ways. In doing so, they test the limits of biomedicine's ultimate promise: the 'gift of life'.

The rhetoric of gift-giving for transplant medicine is explicitly juxtaposed to commodification discourses and contract models of exchange. Influenced by Titmuss's emphasis on altruism, gift-giving has been idealized as a mechanism for fostering the promotion of organs, while preserving and enhancing social life and community values (Titmuss, 1970; Murray, 1996). Its underpinning assumption is that this gift is freely and anonymously given with no expectation or obligation to reciprocate. Indeed, it might be said that organ transplantation, in the context of deceased organ donation, is predicated on maintaining this separation between donor and recipient (Sharp, 2006).

However, anthropological research shows that this is not always possible and, in a similar vein to Mauss, the gifting of organs does not escape the requirements of reciprocity, either implicitly or explicitly (Sharp, 2000; Tutton, 2002). Renee Fox and Judith Swazey (1992) have described the ensuing constricting and mutually fettering obligations that bind giver and receiver as the 'tyranny of the gift', a phrase taken up by many subsequent ethnographic studies of organ donation. Yosuke

Shimazono's (2008) examination of living-related donation in the Philippines illustrates this particular tension by documenting the public and formal ways in which kidney recipients are encouraged to express gratitude. Gifts are generally assumed to flow from adults to children or older to younger siblings, leaving the beneficiary with a debt of varying magnitude. However, as kidneys can be offered in any direction, this particular moral economy is destabilized. Shimazono characterizes the experiences of recipients as a complex mix of gratitude and guilt, which underpins the burden of repaying the gift in some way – financially or by taking responsibility for the donor or the donor's children. For those recipients where obligations to reciprocate are not formally required, Shimazono describes another form of obligation: to be a 'good steward' of the new organ, to keep one's self well. Whatever the mode, reciprocal expectations are complex, persistent and compromising for both donor and recipient.

Studying living-related organ donation in the context of Mexico, Megan Crowley-Matoka's (2005) study shows how the promise of the 'gift of life' fails to achieve its desired-for expectations, something that constitutes a profound paradox in transplant medicine. In Mexico, the social value of a healthy body is revealed through local idioms of production and reproduction, and within the context of family life. Organ transplantation is promoted as the route to resuming a renal patient's productive and reproductive status and bound to a cultural logic of normalcy. As Crowley-Matoka describes, kidney recipients are often unprepared for the realities of living post-transplant. They are caught in perpetual liminality, a 'betwixt and between' state of living with the side-effects of immunosuppressants, the strain of regular medical monitoring and the constant worrying about kidney rejection. Renal recipients are often not healthy enough to return to work, and instead have to negotiate a working life on the fringes of the economy, destabilizing family and reproductive life further.

Conditions such as chronic kidney disease have been acquiring increasing attention as invisible epidemics sweeping throughout countries such as Mexico, disproportionately affecting a poor and 'flexibilized' workforce (Ramirez-Rubio et al., 2013) – a population often in need of healthy organs-for-transplant, while at the same time expected to provide them within the context of family networks (Kierans et al., 2013; Kierans, 2015). Circumstances such as these raise significant questions about the risks attached to living-related organ donation, particularly in places where the likelihood of contracting the disease is substantially higher than the industrialized countries of the Global North. The situation in Mexico, as in many other Latin American countries, is a critical instance of Elliot's bioethical problem as outlined in the introduction: whether we should encourage individuals to willingly harm themselves for the good of another and whether we should encourage individuals to take advantage of another's sacrifice, particularly in the context of poverty and inequality.

In contrast to patients in Mexico and the Philippines, Irish patients are generally recipients of deceased organ donors – what is considered the preferred modality within transplant medicine. Nonetheless, the experiences of kidney recipients in

Ireland carries its own moral weight and picks up elements of both Shimazono's and Crowley-Matoka's arguments. Irish patients, too, experience the 'gift of life' in embodied terms, with consequences for family and wider community relations. They speak of the physical and psychological effects of immunosuppression: their continued sickness; difficulties maintaining a regular working life; difficulties in forming relationships and having a family; difficulties when contemplating an unknown future. For some, a new kidney is readily accommodated within the identity of the organ recipient; for others, it will always retain part of the donor, whose characteristics and personality they may also absorb. That theirs is an organ given by a deceased donor doesn't alter the indebtedness felt by the recipient. Like Shimazono's informants, Irish patients too talk about the importance of being a good steward and the moral and existential pressure to be a grateful patient. While they may publicly espouse and promote the benefits of transplantation, they privately complain about their fear, loneliness and continued experiences of sickness, profoundly aware that no one wants to listen to a transplant recipient complain (Kierans, 2005). Examples such as these demonstrate the problem of relying on overly generalized discourses of gift-giving. Moreover, they also show these discourses to be less a reflection of autonomy and altruism and more the outcome of structured and heavily promoted organ donation campaigns by those institutions with vested interests in the social production of giving (Healy, 2004; Hayden, 2007).

While the juxtaposition between organ givers and receivers often breaks down in practice, it nevertheless continues to hold rhetorical weight as it sustains the mythological promise of organ transplantation. This tendency towards polarizing the mechanisms of exchange has also been employed in the anthropological literature to generate analytical leverage, at times with one side of the exchange equation taking moral precedence over the other, i.e., recipients are often assumed as beneficiaries of the sacrifices others have made (Kierans, 2011).

In Nancy Scheper-Hughes' (2002) well-cited work on the topic, these distinctions take on global proportions. For her, organ givers and organ receivers constitute two unequal populations: 'one socially and medically included, the other excluded, one with and one utterly lacking the ability to draw on the beauty, strength, reproductive, sexual or anatomical power of the other' (Scheper-Hughes, 2002: 4). The former, she continues, are an invisible and discredited collection of anonymous suppliers of spare parts; the latter are cherished patients, 'winners' in the hegemonic narratives spun around transplantation. Recipients, on the other hand, typically feature in her accounts as cyphers: privileged Western consumers juxtaposed with those who through poverty and necessity are forced to sell the organs upon which their health depends.

This iniquitous gap owes much to advances in immunosuppression drug therapy, in particular the drug cyclosporine. Its development has significantly reduced reliance on maintaining genetic similarity through blood and tissue matching, ensuring that more people can serve as kidney donors (Cohen, 2002). The capitalization of immunosuppressants has enabled transplantation to become a global enterprise, with adverse consequences for some of the world's most vulnerable populations.

For Scheper-Hughes, cyclosporine has supported the transfer of organs across the borders of developing and developed countries, moving sick bodies in one direction and healthy bodies in the other (Scheper-Hughes, 2008) in the form of a modern-day biopolitical Kula Ring. In this vein, Scheper-Hughes describes the global traffic in organs, in this much-quoted excerpt, as following the 'modern routes of capital and labour flows [where] organs flow from south to north, from poor to rich, from black and brown to white, and from female to male bodies' (Scheper-Hughes, 2002: 45). While Scheper-Hughes's work has been influential in documenting the injustices and inequalities bound up with the organ trade, it reflects a world too neatly divided and too dependent on an understanding of commodification as a uniform and homogenizing process, one that over-determines the exchange of scarce items such as organs.

Taking and giving 'whole' bodies: from 'gifts of life' to 'gifts of knowledge'

As previously highlighted, there is little doubt that the range of body parts, tissues, cells and genetic materials subject to exchange has expanded exponentially in recent years, in line with the increasing variety of medico-corporate ends to which such parts can be profitably put (Constable, 2009; Moazam et al., 2009). The sheer volume of exchangeable body parts has also and perhaps inevitably increased the demand for whole bodies, with all manner of consequences for the ways in which bodies are appropriated (Lock, 2001; Simpson, 2009). Recent controversies including, for example, that of Biomedical Tissue Services Ltd, the New Jersey tissue bank company found to be 'strip mining' corpses from New York funeral homes to sell on lucrative tissues and bones, have transformed the legendary practice of grave-robbing into its contemporary biotechnical form (Scheper-Hughes, 2006).

While there is much that could be said about the social, cultural and indeed ontological status of the dead body as it is made to work for different interests, I focus, in this last section, on the less prominent, but no less important, issue of 'whole body' procurement. In contrast to the previous examples, I will *not* focus on the therapeutic uses of dead bodies, but instead on their educational capacities – as pedagogical blueprints from which we understand the living body (Sawday, 1995). Again, I suggest that gift-commodity distinctions find little traction here as they continue to overlap and extend each other in all manner of ways. Bodies, living or deceased, following Mary Douglas (1970) and Donna Haraway (1991), are best seen as analogues of society and culture, not only across cultural spaces as the previous sections have marked out but also across historical time (see Chapter 7).

Our point of departure for the body as a knowable medical object is taken from the anatomy courts of fifteenth-century Europe, predominantly through a working relationship between Renaissance artists and the early anatomists whose combined efforts produced an understanding of the structure, function and mechanics of the body (see Chapter 7). The growing corpus of knowledge that anatomy produced over the subsequent centuries was predicated on a ready availability of fresh corpses. As dead bodies were prone to decay, dissections had to be done quickly and were performed in outdoor anatomy courts. The bodies of prisoners, vagrants and the poor largely constituted – to use Cohen's (2004) term – this 'bioavailable' cohort, easily supplied from Europe's expanding urban centres. The anatomizing of human bodies, from Europe's anatomy courts to contemporary medical school environments, has been of great importance to scholars across the natural and social sciences as well as the arts and humanities, with interest focused on the body not only as a site of therapeutic interest but also as a site of artistic, social, cultural, architectural and educational interest.

Against this background, we see that knowledge and value of the body is itself the outcome of embodied practices: the cultural and relational work of anatomy itself – the product of the bodies of the dead and living mutually shaping each other (Hallam, 2010). This is clearly illustrated in Elizabeth Hallam's anthropological and historical work on anatomy in Britain and more specifically on the subject of bones and their articulation. Articulation, advanced by Bruno Latour (2004), attends to the ways in which bodies are jointed and re-jointed in order to obtain a workable human skeleton. It involves a series of practices and technologies to remove flesh, clean and dry bones, as well as ways to order, perforate and reconnect them. Over time, Hallam (2010: 466) shows that descriptions of bones in anatomy must be read within this 'context of practical [and embodied] learning'. Throughout the eighteenth century, she explains, bones used for the purposes of 'skeletopia', i.e., the making of skeletons, were removed from deceased bodies obtained and exchanged through anatomists' social networks – men in positions of medical, military and administrative authority. These networks, she states,

> expanded from locality to colony, facilitating anatomists' collecting and supplying their medical schools with the bodies of the very poor, who died in public institutions and were unclaimed by relatives, as well as the skeletal remains, especially the skulls of indigenous people.
>
> (Hallam, 2010: 480)

Hallam's work shows how the commercial exchange and trafficking of bodies is far from a contemporary concern. Even by the 1780s, the production of skeletons had been commercialized, making full use of the economic cleavages that made it permissible to appropriate the bodies of the poor for the advancement of science. She shows that the articulation of bones, in a similar fashion to the production of blood products, are mutable and unstable in form and substance, at odds 'with notions of bones as durable, as capable of stable longevity, as remains that connect the living with the long dead, the present with the deep past' (Hallam, 2010: 466).

In contrast to the indiscriminate stealing of dead bodies, other modes of procurement might also be said to be bound up with the development of anthropology itself as a 'science of man'. The Societe d'Autopsie Mutuelle (Society of Mutual

Autopsy), based and founded in Paris in 1876, was one of a number of European anthropological associations dedicated to the development of the discipline (Hecht, 2003). Its elite members, which included well-known figures such as Arthur Conan Doyle and Maria Montessori, had pledged their bodies, agreeing to perform autopsies on each other, in the interest of utility and the advancement of knowledge.

Clearly, the donation of bodies for medical science makes much more visible the social relations bound up with both the production of knowledge and the reproduction of bodies as new reified objects. This is also a concern at the heart of Hilary Martinez's work on whole body donation to the Forensic Anthropology Center at Texas State University-San Marcos (FACTS) (Martinez, 2013). The purpose of FACTS is to conduct research on human decomposition processes, the post-mortem interval, human skeletal variation and forensic osteological methods. Facilities such as FACTS came to prominence with the publication of Patricia Cornwall's best-seller *The Body Farm*, based on a precursor to FACTS – the Anthropology Research Facility at the University of Tennessee, Knoxville. Martinez's research enquires into the motivations of those who choose to donate their bodies or those of a loved one to these establishments. Her work demonstrates that whole body donations are not simply driven by an interest in the advancements of science, but are also a much-needed mechanism for those without money to avoid exorbitant funeral costs. Interestingly, this is a gift whose reciprocal reward is returned directly to the giver by way of cost-savings. It is one also where the structural inequalities that characterize dying and disposal (in addition to living) are made indisputably clear. Different types of reciprocal arrangements characterize Hallam's work on the anthropology of anatomy in Britain. Here the emphasis is not financial, but is placed on the importance of memorializing, a practice organized to stress an ethos of dignity and respect and the imperative of gratitude exercised through public memorial services, ceremonies, books of remembrances, plaques and so on (Sharp, 2006; Hallam, 2007).

To some extent, the continued importance of and contemporary organization and administration of whole body donation owes much to the need to circumvent the appropriation or theft of bodies, as discussed earlier. High-profile scandals, such as those concerning the retention of body parts and tissues in the UK,[5] has led to the creation and tightening up of legislation to ensure consent and to control the processes of procurement use and disposal of human tissues and bodies.[6] Nevertheless, the array of materials drawn on for the purposes of anatomy and medical education has increased in recent years. In addition to the use of deceased bodies, some medical schools and institutions work with prosections (preserved body parts), new forms of technological imaging and living body-painting (McLachlan and Patten, 2006; Hallam, 2007), while others work with plastinated prosections purchased from Gunther von Hagens' commercial 'Plastinarium', brought to public attention by the *Korperwelten* or *Body Worlds* exhibition.

Von Hagens' *Body Worlds* has given rise to much debate as to what kind of object the anatomical cadaver is, as well as what the limits of its uses ought to be. *Body Worlds* relies on bodies that are hybridized, a mixture of nature and artifice, achieved through the chemical preservation technique of plastination. This involves immersing the body in formaldehyde to prevent decay. Body fats are removed and fluids are replaced by acetone, which is then replaced by a synthetic resin. The body is either prepared into thin slices and pressed between glass plates or left whole with some parts removed so as to enhance the visibility of others. Von Hagens' corpses are said to be preserved for up to 2,000 years. Many of the bodies used for these purposes have been donated as a result of forms that are handed out to visitors at the exhibition. Von Hagens' critics have raised ethical concerns about the use of donated or gifted bodies for what has been deemed an ambiguous mix of education and entertainment, as well as for explicit commercialization. Others suggest that what von Hagens is doing is no different to what scientists do with living bodies, through the principles of cosmetic surgery (Van Dijck, 2001). Nevertheless, plastination challenges ready-made moralities and further troubles the juxtaposition between the gift and commodity; the real and artificial; nature and culture – binaries I have challenged throughout this chapter (and indeed are challenged throughout this book).

Conclusion

In conclusion, this chapter has shown that gifts, and by extension commodity concepts, while useful in differentiating various modes of exchange, tend to fail us when they are overextended in analyses, particularly when we posit a uniform mechanism underpinning what occurs from one place to another. Neither gifts nor commodities, according to Parry (2008: 1143), can reflect the instability of contemporary modes of exchange or 'our complex, negotiated relations to them'. As I have illustrated, these distinctions are inadequate for the task of explicating the complexities of both contemporary and historical modalities of body exchange.

In contrast to the gift-commodity distinction as a predetermining trope, I have turned attention instead to the ways in which the body and its parts function as sites for enacting various modes of exchange, opening up more nuanced understandings of obligation, interest, entitlement, status, altruism, the desire to contribute to knowledge – scientific and social – and therapeutic wellbeing. In returning to Graham Greene's story, things that can be exchanged, like the exchange of one life for the prospects of another's, have unforeseen and unimagined consequences that are fundamentally social rather than individual in character. Through the processes of giving and receiving, we inevitably work across and create points of intersection between economic, political, cultural and bioethical jurisdictions (Hamdy, 2010; Lundin, 2010; Yea, 2010). This is analytically difficult terrain and to cope with its complexities we must avoid reproducing the polarizing biopolitics that seem internal to it (Kierans, 2011). While the development of anthropology as a discipline has also been bound up with the exchange of bodies and body parts, the challenges that this chapter has outlined, theoretically and methodologically, have relevance far beyond the interests of anthropologists alone.

Notes

1 Anthropologists were in turn building upon earlier political economy traditions, the key expression of which is the work of Karl Marx (see Chapter 4). The political economy tradition has remained a strong one and while it doesn't constitute a discipline in its own right, it draws contributions from across the social sciences to this day. We can see this in the continued relevance of crossover figures such as Karl Polanyi, whose dialogue with Marx involved contributions to anthropology, sociology, economics and social policy, for example. The work of Marshall Sahlins and David Harvey has similarly been taken up across a range of disciplinary fields. The enduring relevance of this tradition has been underscored in the wake of the 2008 financial crisis, where many look beyond or look back to writings on political economy for an analysis. David Graeber's rethinking anthropological accounts of value and exchange possibly stands as the most recent and best-known accounts of this kind.
2 For further work examining the particular types of relations and transformations through which communities attempt to create regimes of value for their reproduction, see Munn (1989).
3 For anthropological research on blood circulations, transactions and transfers, see Copeman (2009a, 2009b) and the 2009 special issue of *Body and Society* on this topic (vol. 15, no. 2).
4 Factor VIII is an essential blood clotting protein, also known as anti-haemophilic factor (AHF). A deficiency of this protein causes one of the main forms of haemophilia.
5 See Redfern and Keeling (2001).
6 See the Human Tissue Act 2004 (England, Wales and Northern Ireland) and also the Human Tissue (Scotland) Act 2006, the Uniform Anatomical Gift Act (USA) and the Odisha Anatomy Act (India).

References

Anagnost, A. (2006) Strange circulations: blood economy in rural China. *Economy and Society*, 34(4): 509–29.

Appadurai, A. (1986) *The Social Life of Things: Commodities in Cultural Perspective*. New York: Cambridge University Press.

Avera, E. (2009) Rationalisation and racialisation in the rainbow nation: inequalities and identity in the South African bone marrow transplant network. *Anthropology and Medicine*, 16: 179–93.

Boas, F. (1888) The Indians of British Columbia. *The Popular Science Monthly*, 32: 636.

Busby, H. (2004) Biobanks, bioethics and concepts of donated blood in the UK. *Sociology of Health and Illness*, 28(6): 850–865.

Callon, M. (1998) *The Laws of the Markets*. Oxford: Blackwell Publishers.

Carsten, J. (2011) Substance and relationality: blood in contexts. *Annual Review of Anthropology*, 40: 19–35.

Cohen, L. (1999) Where it hurts: Indian material for an ethics of organ transplantation. *Daedalus*, 128(4): 135–165.

Cohen, L. (2002) The other kidney: biopolitics beyond recognition. In N. Scheper-Hughes and L. Wacquant (eds.), *Commodifying Bodies*. London: Sage, 9–30.

Cohen, L. (2004) Operability, bioavailability and exception. In A. Ong, and S. Collier (eds.), *Global Assemblages*. Oxford: Blackwell, 79–90.

Cole, D. and Chaikin, I. (1990) *An Iron Hand upon the People: The Law against the Potlatch on the Northwest Coast*. Seattle, WA: University of Washington Press.

Constable, N. (2009). The commodification of intimacy: marriage, sex and reproductive labor. *Annual Review Anthropology*, 38(1): 49–64.
Cooper, M. (2008) *Life as Surplus: Biotechnology and Capitalism in the Neoliberal Era*. Seattle, WA: University of Washington Press.
Copeman, J. (2009a) Introduction: blood donation, bioeconomy, culture. *Body and Society*, 15(2): 1–28.
Copeman, J. (2009b) Gathering points: blood donation and the scenography of 'national integration' in India. *Body and Society*, 15(2): 71–99.
Crowley-Matoka, M. (2005) Desperately seeking 'normal': the promise and perils of living with kidney transplantation. *Social Science and Medicine*, 61(4): 821–831.
Dalsgaard, S. (2007) 'I do it for the chocolate': an anthropological study of blood donation in Denmark. *Distinktion: Scandinavian Journal of Social Theory*, 8(1): 101–115.
Douglas, M. (1970) *Natural Symbols*. London: Barrie & Rockcliff.
Duster, T. (2005) Race and reification in science. *Science*, 307(5712): 1050–1051.
Elliot, C. (1995) Doing harm: living organ donors, clinical research, and the Tenth Man. *Journal of Medical Ethics*, 21: 91–96.
Fausto-Sterling, A. (2008) Race and bones. *Social Studies of Science*, 38(5): 657–694.
Fox, R. and Swazey, J. (1974) *The Courage to Fail: a Social View of Organ Transplants and Dialysis*. Chicago, IL: University of Chicago Press.
Fox, R. and Swazey, J. (1992) *Spare Parts: Organ Replacement in American Society*. New York: Oxford University Press.
Fullwiley, D. (2008) The biologistical construction of race: 'admixture' technology and the new genetic medicine. *Social Studies of Science*, 38(5): 695–735.
Godelier, M. (1999) *The Enigma of the Gift*. Cambridge: Polity Press.
Gordon, E. (2002) What 'race' cannot tell us about access to kidney transplantation. *Cambridge Quarterly of Healthcare Ethics*, 11: 134–141.
Graeber, D. (2001) *Toward an Anthropological Theory of Value: The False Coin of Our Own Dreams*. New York: Palgrave.
Greene, G. (1985). *The Tenth Man*. London: The Bodley Head and Anthony Blond.
Gregory, C. (1982) *Gifts and Commodities*. London: Academic Press.
Hallam, E. (2007) Anatomical bodies and materials of memory. In B. Brooks-Gordon, F. Ebtehaj, J. Herring, M.H. Johnson and M. Richards (eds.), *Death Rites and Rights*, Oxford: Hart Publishing, 279–298.
Hallam, E. (2010) Articulating bones: an epilogue. *Journal of Material Culture*, 15(4): 465–492.
Hamdy, S. (2010) The organ transplant debate in Egypt: a social anthropological analysis. *Droit et Cultures*, 59: 357–365.
Haraway, D. (1991) *Simians, Cyborgs and Women: the Reinvention of Nature*. New York: Routledge.
Hayden, C. (2007) Taking as giving: bioscience, exchange, and the politics of benefit-sharing. *Social Studies of Science*, 37(5): 729–758.
Healy, K. (2004) Altruism as an organizational problem: the case of organ procurement. *American Sociological Review*, 69: 387–404.
Hecht, J. (2003) *The End of the Soul: Scientific Modernity, Atheism and Anthropology in France, 1876–1936*. New York: Columbia University Press.
Hogle, L. (1999) *Recovering the Nation's Body: Cultural Memory, Medicine and the Politics of Redemption*. New Brunswick, NJ: Rutgers University Press.
Johansen, D. (1967) *Empire of the Columbia: A History of the Pacific Northwest*, 2nd edn. New York: Harper & Row.
Kierans, C. (2005) Narrating kidney disease: the significance of sensation and time in the emplotment of patient experience. *Culture, Medicine and Psychiatry*, 29: 341–359.

Kierans, C. (2011) Anthropology, organ transplantation and the immune system: Resituating commodity and gift exchange. *Social Science and Medicine*, 73: 1469–1476.

Kierans, C. (2015) Biopolitics and capital: poverty, mobility and the body-in-transplantation in Mexico. *Body and Society*, early view form.

Kierans, C. and Cooper, J. (2011) Organ donation, genetics, race and culture. *Anthropology Today*, 27(6): 11–14.

Kierans, C., Padilla-Altamira, C., Garcia-Garcia, G., Ibarra-Hernandez, M. and Mercado, F.J. (2013) When health systems are barriers to health care: challenges faced by Mexican kidney patients, *PLOS ONE*, 8(10): 1–7.

Laidlaw, J. (2000) A free gift makes no friends. *Journal of the Royal Anthropological Institute*, 6(4): 617–634.

Latour, L. (2004) How to talk about the body? The normative dimension of science studies. *Body and Society*, 10(2–3): 205–229.

Lederer, S. (2008) *Flesh and Blood: Organ Transplantation and Blood Transfusion in Twentieth-Century America*. Oxford: Oxford University Press.

Lévi-Strauss, C. (1969 [1949]) *The Elementary Structures of Kinship*. Translated by J.H. Bell and J.R. von Sturmer. Boston, MA: Beacon Press.

Lock, M. (2001) *Twice Dead: Organ Transplants and the Reinvention of Death*. Berkeley, CA: University of California Press.

Lundin, S.M. (2010). Organ economy: organ trafficking in Moldova and Israel. *Public Understanding of Science*, 1: 1–16.

Malinowski, B. (1922) *Argonauts of the Western Pacific*. Oxon: Routledge.

Marcus, G. (1998) *Ethnography through Thick and Thin*. Princeton, NJ: Princeton University Press.

Martinez, H. (2013) *'I Don't Need It, You Can Have It': Motivations for Whole Body Donation*. Master's Dissertation. Department of Anthropology, Texas State University.

Mauss, M. (1967) *The Gift: Forms and Functions of Exchange in Archaic Societies*. New York: Norton Library and Routledge & Kegan Paul Ltd.

McLachlan, J. and Patten, D. (2006) Anatomy teaching: ghosts of the past, present and future. *Medical Education*, 40(3): 243–253.

Moazam, F, Zaman, R.M. and Jafarey, A.M. (2009) Conversations with kidney vendors in Pakistan: an ethnographic study. *Hastings Center Report*, 39(3): 29–44.

Munn, N. (1989) *The Fame of Gawa: A Symbolic Study of Value Transformation in a Massim Society*. Durham, NC: Duke University Press.

Murray, T. (1996) Organ vendors, families and the gift of life. In S. Younger, R. Fox and L. O'Connell (eds.), *Organ Transplantation: Meanings and Realities*. Madison, WI: University of Wisconsin Press, 101–125.

Nash, J. (1979) *We Eat the Mines and the Mines Eat Us: Dependency and Exploitation in Bolivian Tin Mines*. Chicago, IL: University of Chicago Press.

Parry, B. (2008) Entangled exchange: reconceptualising the characterisation and practice of bodily commodification. *Geoform*, 39: 1133–1144.

Parry, J. (1986) The gift, the Indian gift and the 'Indian gift'. *Man*, 21(3): 466–469.

Ramirez-Rubio, O., McClean, M.D., Amador, J.J. and Brooks, D.R. (2013) An epidemic of chronic kidney disease in Central America: an overview. *Journal of Epidemiology and Community Health*, 67: 1–3.

Reddy, D. (2007) Good gifts for the common good: blood and bioethics in the market for genetic research. *Cultural Anthropology*, 22(3): 429–472.

Redfern, M. and Keeling, J. (2001) *The Royal Liverpool Children's Inquiry Report (The Redfern Report)*. London: Stationery Office.

Robertson, J. (2002) Blood talks: eugenic modernity and the creation of new Japanese. *History and Anthropology*, 13(3): 191–216.

Sahlins, M. (1963) Poor man, rich man, big man, chief: political types in Melanesia and Polynesia. *Comparative Studies in Society and History*, 15(3): 285–303.

Sahlins, M. (1972) *Stone Age Economics*. Oxfordshire: Routledge.

Sawday, J. (1995) *The Body Emblazoned: Dissection and the Human Body in Renaissance Culture*. New York: Routledge.

Scheper-Hughes, N. (2000) The global traffic in human organs. *Current Anthropology*, 41(2): 191–224.

Scheper-Hughes, N. (2002) Commodity fetishism in organs trafficking. In N. Scheper-Hughes and L. Wacquant (eds.), *Commodifying Bodies*, London: Sage, 31–62.

Scheper-Hughes, N. (2006) Alistair Cooke's bones. *Anthropology Today*, 22(6): 10–15.

Scheper-Hughes, N. (2008) The last commodity. *Dissenting Knowledges*, Pamplet Series, 6: 1–55.

Shao, J. (2006) Fluid labor and blood money: the economy of HIV/AIDS in rural Central China. *Cultural Anthropology*, 21(4): 535–569.

Shao, J. and Scoggin, M. (2009) Solidarity and distinction in blood: contamination, morality and variability. *Body and Society*, 15(2): 29–49.

Sharp, L. (2000) The commodification of the body and its parts. *Annual Review of Anthropology*, 29: 287–328.

Sharp, L. (2001) Commodified kin: death, mourning and competing claims on the bodies of organ donors in the United States. *American Anthropologist*, 103: 1–21.

Sharp, L. (2006) *Strange Harvest: Organ Transplants, Denatured Bodies, and the Transformed Self*. Berkeley, CA: University of California Press.

Shimazono, Y. (2008) Repaying and cherishing the gift of life: gift exchange and living related kidney transplantation in the Philippines. *Anthropology in Action*, 15(3): 34–46.

Simpson, B. (2009) 'Please give a drop of blood': blood donation, conflict and the haemato-global assemblage in contemporary Sri Lanka. *Body and Society*, 15: 101–122.

Strathern, A. (1974) *Ongka's Big Moka: The Kawelka of Papua New Guinea*. Directed by C. Nairn. Great Britain: *Disappearing World* Series.

Strathern, M. (1988) *The Gender of the Gift: Problems with Women and Problems with Society in Melanesia*. Berkeley, CA: University of California Press.

Taussig, M. (1980) *The Devil and Commodity Fetishism*. Charlotte, NC: University of North Carolina Press.

Thomas, N. (1991) *Entangled Objects: Exchange, Material Culture, and Colonialism in the Pacific*. Cambridge, MA: Harvard University Press.

Titmuss, R. (1970) *The Gift Relationship: From Human Blood to Social Policy*. Edited by A. Oakley and J. Ashton. London: London School of Economics.

Tutton, R. (2002) Gift relationships in genetics research. *Science as Culture*, 11(4): 523–542.

Van Dijck, J. (2001) Bodyworlds: the art of plastinated cadavers. *Configurations*, 9(1): 99–126.

Waldby, C. and Mitchell, R. (2006) *Tissue Economies: Blood, Organs, and Cell Lines in Late Capitalism*. Durham, NC: Duke University Press.

Weiner, A. (1992) *Inalienable Possessions: The Paradox of Keeping-while-Giving*. Berkeley, CA: University of California Press.

Wolf, E. (1982) *Europe and the People without History*. Berkeley, CA: University of California Press.

Yea, S. (2010). Trafficking in part(s): the commercial kidney market in a Manila slum, Philippines. *Global Social Policy*, 10(3): 358–376.

7

THE BODY

Ciara Kierans and Kirsten Bell

> The body is thus not a provisional residence of something superior – an immortal soul, the universal or thought – but what leaves a dynamic trajectory by which we learn to register and become sensitive to what the world is made of. Such is the great virtue of this definition: there is no sense in defining the body directly, but only in rendering the body sensitive to what these other elements are. By focusing on the body, one is immediately – or rather, mediately – directed to what the body has become aware of.
>
> Bruno Latour, 'How to talk about the body?'

Introduction

In the course of the previous chapters, we have each shown how six concepts – culture, society, magic, production, kinship and exchange – have been taken up for different ends across the social and natural sciences. We have done so with reference to a series of examples that have helped to demonstrate that these concepts provide powerful tools for analysing phenomena that sit at the intersections between medicine, science and technology: i.e., the use and exchange of blood and tissues; the pervasive problem of cancer and the consequences of the 'new genetics'; and the complex and shifting biotechnical terrain of fertility and birth. In this, our final chapter, we turn to an implicit presence in all previous chapters: the body, or more specifically, 'the embodied subject'.

What is most interesting about reflection on 'the body', which is not strictly a concept in its own right, is that it has led to conceptual innovation and the proliferation of new concepts across many fields of research (e.g., embodiment, biopolitics, performativity and so on). Work on the body has given rise to multiple forms of understanding, organization and practice, which, in turn, link our everyday lives as individuals to wider collectivities (families, communities, populations, institutions, polities and nations). In other words, we read the body as productive of ways of thinking and doing, as well as produced by ways of thinking and doing.[1] This is equally true of the social and natural sciences, generating in both cases a vast array of scholarship examining all aspects of bodily life.[2] Thus, of all the concepts we explore in this book, 'the body' has been the most extensively worked on as a conceptual site.

Because of the breadth and depth of scholarship on this topic, and its ambiguous status as a concept per se, our approach therefore departs somewhat from the previous chapters. In particular, we do not attempt to provide an historical account of scholarship on the body; instead, we focus on three conceptual frames that enable us to map the ways in which studies of the body establish connections across biology, society and culture, namely: lived bodies, disciplined bodies and classified bodies. Echoing Scheper-Hughes and Lock (1987: 7), our account thus presents something of a partial and fragmentary 'personal itinerary through paths of inquiry we believe to hold particular promise for theory building and further research'. While this approach has enabled us to tell a more coherent story about 'the body' (or rather 'bodies'), it has inevitably meant that certain key contributions to scholarship in this area have been downplayed. For example, although we have incorporated a range of feminist thinkers and their work throughout the chapter, we have not provided an explicit section on feminist scholarship on the body, although this is an area that has produced vital contributions to the social sciences more broadly as well as to theorizing the body.[3]

We begin our account with a brief historical overview of the body in and of medical science – the normative conventional body seen as a discrete, material, 'brute fact of nature' (Csordas, 1994: 1) – before proceeding to a discussion of the three conceptual frames identified above.[4] 'Lived bodies' focuses on theorists that start from the embodied character of everyday life: the ways in which the body is confronted in a direct, immediate and personal way, as in pain, sickness, harm, injury and pleasure. 'Disciplined bodies' encompasses scholarship that articulates the particular and situated ways in which bodies are worked on and organized socially and culturally – in other words, the framework within which individuals as embodied subjects are formed. Finally, 'classified bodies' characterizes approaches that situate the body as the locus of identity – something that incorporates examinations of how institutions (such as medicine) inculcate and reinforce group identification. Work here points to a wider social infrastructure within which individuals are organized and, in turn, governed on much broader national and international scales: the terrain of biopolitics. Importantly, each of these ways of framing the body facilitates a critical dialogue, one in which it is possible to rethink nature–culture, mind–body and subject–object boundaries and divides. Finally, we close with a case study on the rise of neuroscientific approaches to addiction as a way of illustrating the kinds of insights afforded by a focus on the 'three bodies'.

Situating 'natural bodies'

A persistent challenge for social and cultural theorists of the body is countering the dominance of what Donna Haraway (1991) calls the 'universalized natural body' as the archetype for objectified scientific discourse. *This* body, routinely portrayed as a fact of nature, has been so embedded in our imaginations that it's difficult to envision any aspect of the human condition being debated today without recourse or reference to its particular material configurations. Emerging out of – and essentialized through – the practices and discourses of scientific medicine, written accounts of what constitutes the body and its functions in Western societies can be traced back to the Greeks and the work of the physician and anatomist Galen of Pergamon. Galen's work was subsequently taken up and transmitted by Islamic physicians in the Middle Ages, before being reinterpreted and re-codified in the anatomy courts of sixteenth- and seventeenth-century Europe (Porter, 2003).

It is within this historical context and through the close working relationships between anatomists and artists that we see the emergence of the body as a proper subject for science, something whose operations, mechanics and secrets could be made known through systematic inquiry (see also Chapter 6). Prior to the sixteenth century, human dissections were rare, with knowledge of the body's internal workings largely a product of the classical imagination, extrapolated from animal dissections and ordered through categories of cosmology and theology (Sawday, 1995). Work of this kind relied on much the same idea of the body advanced by Plato. For Plato, the body was mere matter of flesh: imperfect, earthly and time-bound. The soul, on the other hand, was perfect, heavenly and timeless. Truth was only to be found in the contemplation of the latter. The work of dissection not only broke with such conceptions, but also with one of the oldest Western taboos by transgressing the sanctity of the dead body. Dissection challenged the classical binaries of body and soul, while marking out new sites of tension: those between body and mind. This shift from a metaphysics of the body to a mechanics or science of the body would be driven further by a new generation of philosophers, *inter alia* Bacon, Descartes, Gassendi, Boyle and Newton, and graphically exhibited through representations of the body in Renaissance art (Porter, 2003).

The foremost example of artistic contributions to this emerging area of science is Leonardo da Vinci's studiously observed and intricately detailed drawings of the interior workings of the human body (Sawday, 1995). In the course of more than 20 years of study, da Vinci dissected more than 19 corpses, not only visually depicting the body in the context of its viscera, but the vital relationship between the parts and the whole. According to Porter, these studies of the body in motion prompted a new research programme in anatomy, physiology and medicine, one in which investigators came to view the body as a '*machina carnis*, a machine of the flesh' (Porter, 2003: 51).

Da Vinci's work graphically illustrates the new approaches and methods of the natural sciences, exemplifying the importance of observation – here through dissection – as central to the production of new truths and laws. The anatomized body was not simply a potent object of and for knowledge; it was also a potent symbol of its age. As the established canons of sixteenth-century thought were pulled apart and discredited, so too were the wider institutions and authority structures in which they were embedded. Across the arts, humanities and sciences, the mind, the state, the economy and society would find their own places as new objects of concern within the emerging discourses of psychology, politics, economics and sociology. But few would exert the same fascination or were granted as much importance as the body. Best captured by Hobbes' *Leviathan*, the body and 'man, himself' became the 'measure of all things': a key site for forging radically new ways of thinking about and organizing human life, starting from the organic individual and working up and out to the state (Hobbes, 2012 [1651]).

According to Michel Foucault (1978), this new knowledge of the body and the new bodies of knowledge its study gave rise to characterized the emergence of a recognizably modern (as opposed to ancient) episteme, one in which understandings of 'man' were reconstructed around a new set of tensions. These tensions, while shaped by the shift from metaphysical knowledge (religious, philosophical, supernatural) to scientific knowledge (grounded in empirical observations), are further complicated by a process that Foucault, in a reworking of Kant, refers to as the creation of an 'empiricio-transcendental doublet' (Foucault, 1970: 321). This 'doublet', or doubling, refers to the body/'man' not only as the subject *and* object of knowledge, but also paradoxically as the agent or generator of this knowledge – 'the organiser of the spectacle in which he appears' (Dreyfus and Rabinow, 1983: 29). According to Foucault, the scientific body – as one of the cornerstones of scientific thinking – could no longer simply be reduced to the category of nature, ordered and organized by the cosmos, but instead explained according to its own internal laws and operations by those who looked at nature from the outside (the 'god' view). As commentators then and since well understood, this would leave no place for society, culture and the complexities of subjectivity and difference. Attempts to reduce the body to its mechanics alone therefore suppressed the body's social and cultural moorings. At the same time, attempts to privilege those social and cultural moorings ran the risk of abandoning the body's materiality (Butler, 1993).

These Cartesian distinctions, often employed in the interest of preserving different orders of knowledge, had produced an unbridgeable chasm. How to understand this chasm – the relationship between nature and society, the knower and the known – has remained a perennial problem.[5] As Scheper-Hughes and Lock observe:

> We lack a precise vocabulary with which to deal with mind-body-society interactions and so are left suspended in hyphens, testifying to the disconnectedness of our thoughts. We are forced to resort to such fragmented concepts as the bio-social, the psycho-somatic, the somato-social as altogether feeble ways of expressing the myriad ways in which the mind speaks through the body, and the ways in which society is inscribed on the expectant canvas of human flesh.
>
> (Scheper-Hughes and Lock, 1987: 10)

In the sections that follow, we keep these tensions firmly in view, tracing three interconnected ways of *re*framing the subject/object division that derive from contemporary approaches to the study of the body as at once a biological, existential, social and cultural phenomenon.

Lived bodies: the elemental site of experience

We start with work that takes up the experience of being *in* a body – or being embodied – and how we confront that directly. Taking Elaine Scarry's influential writing as our starting point, we draw attention to what happens when pain throws our embodiment into relief and makes our bodies profoundly present to us (Leder, 1990). We will subsequently show how pain's effects trouble subject–object relations, drawing on phenomenology and the embodiment paradigm to highlight not just the body's inseparability from the world in which it is enmeshed, but also the ways in which the world changes for changed bodies.

In *A Body in Pain*, Scarry (1985) reflects on the arresting immediacy of the experience of pain and the profound ways in which pain intensifies the status of the body-in-the-world. For Scarry, as well as for others who have written on the subject (Schutz, 1971; DelVecchio Good et al., 1994; Jackson, 1994), pain is, in essence, non-dualistic. Occurring simultaneously inside and outside oneself, pain

> [i]s a pure physical experience of negation; an immediate sensory rendering of 'against', of something being against one, and of something one must be against. Even though it occurs within oneself, it is at once identified as 'not oneself', 'not me'.
>
> (Scarry, 1985: 52)

Consequently, we talk about pain as an 'it' hurting me, rather than an 'I' hurting. By extension, pain is simultaneously a bodily and mental-emotional experience. It challenges the boundaries between the interior and exterior worlds that mark out the territories of self and other, private and public, subject and object. In doing so, pain fatally undermines the Cartesian mind–body dualism. Furthermore, its status is prior to language and objectification. Outside of metaphors and metonyms, pain can only be expressed through a pre-symbolic language of cries and shrieks (Scarry, 1985: 5). After all, bodily experiences, as Maurice Merleau-Ponty (1962) observes, do not begin as objects to or for us; rather, they end up as such.

Merleau-Ponty provides one set of resources for thinking about the issues raised by Scarry's discussion of pain, particularly in his attempts to provide a framework that captures the ways in which changes in our bodies manifest our being-in-the-world. Building on the legacy of phenomenologists such as Husserl, Heidegger, Sartre and others, Merleau-Ponty advocates a paradigm of 'embodiment' as a non-dualistic resource to reconcile bodies, selves and society. His point of departure is straightforward: we do not experience a world that society and culture are external to; our concrete, embodied experience is social and cultural from the start. Society and culture are conditions of bodily experience, but our embodiment is simultaneously the ground of society and culture. In consequence, neither side can be meaningfully considered in isolation. As Merleau-Ponty puts it,

> It is as false to place ourselves in society as an object among other objects, as it is to place society within ourselves as an object of thought and in both cases the mistake lies in treating the social as an object. We must return to the social with which we are in contact by the mere fact of existing and which we carry about inseparably with us before objectification.
>
> (Merleau-Ponty, 1962: 362)

This orientation to the body as lived – neither reducibly material nor social alone – has enjoyed growing influence in the social sciences in recent decades. The anthropologist Thomas Csordas, in drawing together the work of Merleau-Ponty, Bourdieu and Mauss (who we pick up in the following section), argues explicitly for the body as the locus or existential ground for culture and society. He defines the body 'as our first and most natural instrument, the wellspring of our existence, one with a history that behaves in new ways at particular historical moments' (Csordas, 1994: 1). And in this, following Merleau-Ponty's lead, he distinguishes between studies of *embodiment* and studies of the *body* as a 'discrete organic entity' separated from society and culture (Csordas, 1994: 12).

The work of Jonathan Miller (2000) in *The Body in Question* provides a practical illustration of the value of this distinction. A neurologist working at the intersections of medicine, the humanities and the arts, Miller distinguishes what he refers to as the *felt* body from the *object* body. He asks us to imagine if the body we see is the body we immediately feel, suggesting that if we close our eyes and think of our own shape, what we feel is unlike what we see. Miller's felt body is that which allows us to grasp our physical existence in the world, while at the same time distinguishing the world from us. Drawing from his work with people who have suffered a stroke, Miller shows the ways in which this felt body can become impaired – impairments that profoundly reconfigure the stroke sufferer's relationship to the world. As a consequence, he talks about the felt body becoming one-sided or partialized, evidenced by the tendency among some stroke patients to put gloves on only one hand, failing to recognize the other as part of the self. Miller's neurological work demonstrates the central significance of embodied experience to our practical ways of navigating the world. Bodily change, in this case through damage to the brain and its functions, profoundly reconfigures the world around us – what the world *is* and *can be* – because of change to our embodiment.

We gain still further insights from work that examines the technological *extension* of bodies, notably through the concept of the 'cyborg' – a hybrid of human and machine, the natural and the technological (Haraway, 1991; Casper, 1995; Dumit, 1995; Hables Gray, 2002). Hybrid or cyborg bodies have been considered by some to be new forms of threat to an otherwise embodied and sovereign self (Young,

1997). For others, however, they represent new possibilities for living (Haraway, 1991).[6] In a return to Marx,[7] Haraway, the central figure in this area of research, points out that we are all creoles, all cyborgs, of different sorts and this has both positive and negative implications. In contemporary medicine, cyborgs emerge from a wide range of biotechnical interventions: prostheses, imaging technologies and implantable devices, alongside technologically aided ways of seeing, screening, testing, transplanting, researching and so on (Davis-Floyd, 1994; Casper, 1995). Whatever the source of transformation, Haraway contends that we need not be afraid of these permanently partial identities or contradictory standpoints. They reveal the particular conditions – social, political, economic and technical – which ground our experiences in and of the world and reveal the ways in which bodies are socialized and embodied subjects are formed.

Trained bodies: disciplining subjects

When it comes to thinking about the enrolment of the lived body in society and culture, Mauss's classic essay, 'The techniques of the body' (1934), had a decisive influence on subsequent theorizing the body. Following the analytical line set down by Émile Durkheim (see Chapter 2), Mauss asserted that it was only through the social that physiological and psychological matters found expression. His contention was that bodily practices and expressions – from cries to words, gestures to rituals – could be, indeed *were*, read as signs and symbols. As *translations*, they made evident the presence of a group or society – those for whom the experience was being translated. Just as for Merleau-Ponty there can be no asocial experience, for Mauss, there can be no such thing as asocial behaviour. Every bodily action contained within it the imprint of socialization, from how we sit to how we walk, run, throw a ball and so on. To illustrate, Mauss referred to the variation in digging practices found within the trenches of World War I. He explained:

> During the War, I was able to make many observations on this specificity of [bodily] techniques, in particular, the technique of *digging*. The English troops I was with did not know how to use French spades, which forced us to change 8,000 spades when we relieved a French division, and vice versa. This plainly shows that a manual knack can only be learnt slowly. Every technique properly so-called has its own form.
>
> (Mauss, 1992 [1934]: 457)

To emphasize bodily practice as a learned and patterned set of arrangements, Mauss used the term 'habitus', defining it as 'prestigious imitation': the process through which individuals learn the social language for expressing their thoughts, emotions and physical experience. In other words, Mauss showed the ways in which individual bodily practices are turned into shared social facts, as individuals are 'trained' and learn how to do (and to feel and think) as others do. Bodily practice, for Mauss, was the point where Durkheim's 'collective consciousness' came to be effectively and durably instilled. However, as Merleau-Ponty (1964) has observed, Mauss's way of making contact with the social exhibited some subtle but important differences from Durkheim's view. Merleau-Ponty pointed out that Durkheim's view of the social constrained it to the 'psychical', treating it as external to the individual. It therefore lacked 'a patient penetration of its object, communication with it' (Merleau-Ponty, 1964: 115). In Merleau-Ponty's view, Mauss overcame this dichotomy because social facts were now 'inserted into the depths of the individual' (1964: 115). In effect, Mauss developed an analytic frame that no longer forced scholars to choose between the individual and the collective – the collective (society) was imprinted in the individual and vice versa.

The intellectual debts to Mauss's work are perhaps most explicit in Pierre Bourdieu's influential reworking of the concept of 'habitus' (see Chapter 2). According to Bourdieu, 'habitus' refers to:

> Structured structures, generative principles of distinct and distinctive practices – what the worker eats, and especially the way he eats it, ... habitus are also structuring structures, different classifying schemes, classification principles, different principles of vision and division, different tastes. Habitus make different differences; they implement distinctions between what is good and what is bad, what is right and what is wrong.
>
> (Bourdieu, 1996: 17)

In other words, habitus reflects, 'the way society becomes deposited in persons in the form of lasting dispositions, or trained capacities' (Wacquant cited in Navarro, 2006: 16). While Bourdieu also attempts, in part, to bridge aspects of subjectivism and objectivism, his orientation is an account of habitus in which it is largely determined by the structures of culture and society.[8] His thinking shares commonalities with other foundational and broadly structural accounts of the body in anthropology, especially Mary Douglas's (1966, 1973) emphasis on the body as an analogue of social and cultural formations. For Douglas (1973: 93): 'The social body constrains the way the physical body is perceived. The physical experience of the body, always modified by the social categories through which it is known, sustains a particular view of society.' Thus, a focus on the body enables us to understand how different social and cultural groups demarcate the world around a system of categorical binaries including, for example, the poles of 'purity and danger' (Douglas, 1966).

Moving beyond perspectives grounded more directly in structuralist traditions, we find a different sort of attempt to consider the historically particular and spatially sited ways in which bodies come to be trained in the work of Foucault. Employing a genealogical approach, Foucault searches out comparative instances that show how and when power comes to be bound up with the body's functions and practices – revealing the body not just to be a site where power is inscribed but where it is harnessed as a conduit for power's further exercise.

Foucault argues that ways of imprinting or training individuals became more explicit in the processes of institutionalization at play throughout the nineteenth century, which worked to break down bodily practices into component elements. One way he illustrates this is by examining the body as its shifts from an object to subject of punishment, which Foucault marks out through the transition from the public execution to the rise of the prison system. In the opening sections of *Discipline and Punish*, Foucault (1975) describes the public execution of 'Damiens' in 1757, detailing how the executioner sets about his torture: tearing away the pieces of Damiens' flesh, repeatedly aggravating his wounds, over which are poured a boiling potion, before Damiens' body is dismembered limb by limb.

The public spectacle of punishment is contrasted with the daily round of activities that characterize life for the prison inmate about a century later: the regimented ordering and time-tabling of work, washing, bed-making, eating, praying and so on (Foucault, 1975). In the time period between these typical scenes of punishment: 'the spectacle of the scaffold' and 'the time-table', the body, no longer the target of punishment, becomes its instrument or intermediary.[9] We see the body of Damiens being individualized and made exterior to society, in contrast to the prisoner, whose body is completely socialized, invested by power and organized towards the performance of different tasks. Punishment has become what Foucault calls 'an economy of suspended rights'. Charged with administering the body under these conditions, the prison generates a new range of personnel, removing the duty of punishment from the executioner and replacing it with the work of welfare, education and reform, administered by doctors, warders, chaplains, educationalists and so on.

The modern prison system situates the body within a political economy, one in which power develops its justifications, rules, knowledges and discourses in and through the body by probing it, marking it, training it, torturing it and making it productive in very specific ways. Doing so depends on a knowledge of the body beyond its structures and functions: it involves a knowledge and mastery of its entire capacities so that they are made 'docile' and put to productive use. This political technology of the body shows power not as something possessed but as a strategy, what Foucault refers to as a 'micro-physics of power'. From the nineteenth century onwards, this micro-physics of power came to characterize the organization of bodies within the disciplinary spaces of hospitals, prisons, factories, schools, army barracks, etc.

Although coming at the same problem from different angles, Erving Goffman's *Asylums* (1961) can be profitably read alongside Foucault's *Discipline and Punish* (1975). Whereas Foucault takes an historical approach to the emergence of a set of techniques centred on the body and their diffusion across a range of institutional sites, Goffman draws on a set of first-hand descriptions in conjunction with the biographical writings of those who have been processed through what he calls 'total institutions', e.g., prisons, army barracks, psychiatric hospitals, convents and ships. He goes on to discuss the techniques that work to break down not only bodily practice, but individuality, such as those of surveillance and control – systems typically described, after Foucault, as 'panoptic'. These techniques work to curtail the free expression of the self, and reshape people into standardized, institutionally tractable types: inmates, the mentally ill, soldiers, nuns and sailors.

The next section takes up these broader constituencies or collectivities to examine the kinds of subject positions that emerge out of the disciplinary techniques described above. In particular, we focus on the classificatory apparatuses that work to buttress such subject positions by establishing patterns of consequential similarity and difference through distinctions that facilitate the government of bodies. These, in turn, establish the parameters within which population welfare and health, for example, are organized and administered.

Classified bodies: the architecture of government

We start this section by returning to the work of Emily Martin, featured in Chapter 4. Martin's (1987) genealogy of women's reproductive lives shows how their bodily experiences have been (re)organized in and through the disciplinary practices of obstetric and gynaecological medicine as a particular site for intervention. Concerned with the active management of birth as an event subdivided into a series of stages and sub-stages, we see in obstetrics the reflection of contemporary industrial production systems mediated through the technology of forceps, foetal imaging devices and pharmacological supports. Observed from this standpoint, the female body has been made manipulable – capable of being acted upon – by approaching it as an analogue of productive systems, of which the manufacturing process is an archetype. Obstetric medicine thus shows the body to be embedded within a political field, but one, importantly, also structured by assumptions of pathology and risk. Reproduction is not simply productive of childbirth; it also typically gives rise to a particular type of gendered subjectivity, one that is fragmented, lacking autonomy and organized by forces beyond the control of women (Martin, 1987). While women's reproductive processes constitute a particular disciplinary terrain that reconstructs and classifies women's bodies and subjectivity, ways of representing women's bodies also imply possibilities for medical interventions, and in many respects, are predicated on them.[10] It is the practice of classification – more specifically, the practice of classifying bodies – and the implications that follow from it that provide the focus of this section.

The significance of classification for the production of bodily subjects – as bodily subjects of particular kinds – is something we have already touched upon in previous chapters. The category 'BME' (black and minority ethnic), for example, as described in Chapter 1, has clearly emerged from ways of inscribing genetic difference, sickness and inequality onto the bodies of those who are to be defined by their race and/or ethnicity. In the context of transplant medicine, this has been shown to produce a particular 'species' of kidney recipient and a particular 'species' of kidney donor: both defined by their minority ethnic status and consequent obligations and responsibilities.

Classifying or labelling is one moment within what Foucault (1978: 60) calls the 'constitution of subjects'. To explicate their constitution or construction, he suggests:

> We should try to discover how it is that subjects are gradually, progressively, really and materially constituted through a multiplicity of organisms, forces, energies, materials, desires, thoughts, etc. We should try to grasp subjection in its material instance as a constitution of subjects.
>
> (Foucault, 1980: 97)

As classifications and the subject matter they construct often end up as taken-for-granted, ostensibly inevitable or 'natural' facts of the world, it is important to identify how they come to be produced. Ian Hacking (2000) suggests that we pay attention to the 'matrixes': the wider contexts, infrastructures and practices within which classifications or constructs acquire their significance.[11] The key point to note here is that classificatory devices, particularly those which have been naturalized (e.g., motherhood or race), are always situated and contingent features of our social worlds. To give an example on the constitution of identity, Haraway explains,

> I am conscious of the odd perspective provided by my historical position – a PhD in biology for an Irish Catholic girl was made possible by Sputnik's impact on US national science education policy. I have a body and mind as much constructed by the post-Second World War arms race and cold war as by the women's movements.
>
> (Haraway, 1991: 173)

Haraway argues for a permanent partiality and fluidity to the production of selves, bodies and 'species' of individuals. The classificatory apparatuses that hold them in place are, after all, moving targets subject to manipulation and change, via what Hacking (2006) refers to as various 'engines of discovery'. These engines – the methods we use to gain purchase on the objects of our interests – in turn, 'make up people':

> Statistical analysis of classes of people is a fundamental engine. We constantly try to medicalise: doctors tried to medicalise suicide as early as the 1830s. The brains of suicides were dissected to find the hidden cause. More generally, we try to biologise, to recognise a biological foundation for the problems that beset a class of people. More recently, we have hoped to geneticise as much as possible. Thus obesity, once regarded as a problem of incontinence, or weakness of the will, becomes the province of medicine, then of biology, and at present we search for inherited genetic tendencies.
>
> (Hacking, 2006: 24)

Further examples have been presented in the other chapters of this book, including the ways that the practice of ethnography and the theories that accompanied it often produced those it seeks to study as artefacts of its interests, e.g., the kinship system of the Yapese (Chapter 5) and Sahlins' 'big men' (Chapter 6). As classifications become established and institutionalized, their uses, functions and consequences acquire greater stability (see Chapters 2 and 4). In *Sorting Things Out: Classification and its Consequences*, Geoffrey Bowker and Susan Leigh Star (1999) show classification systems to be ubiquitous artefacts of history and politics, an achievement of the work of the modern bureaucratic state. The functions performed by classifications are indispensable. They enable communication across different contexts, producing an ecology of formal and informal arrangements that are made to meet the needs of heterogeneous communities – some cooperative and some coercive (Bowker and Star, 1999).

There are countless examples of how such classificatory systems work across health and medical arenas. Hacking's (2013) discussion of the American Psychiatric Association's *Diagnostic and Statistical Manual of Mental Disorders* (DSM) provides an excellent illustration – one that is especially pertinent to our case study on addiction below. Establishing the criteria for a taxonomy of mental illness, following alterations to the DSM over time not only provides a way of tracing how mental health categories come to be made and remade, but also shows how they work to calibrate the boundaries between the normal and the pathological. Now in its fifth iteration, the DSM has seen what were once termed 'disorders', such as menstrual dysphoric disorder or homosexuality, declassified while others have been refined and consolidated, such as autism spectrum disorders (Regier et al., 2013). Being assigned a DSM code has powerful consequences, particularly within the USA. It can determine what kind of treatments a patient has access to and, indeed, whether their health insurance will pay. It can shape how patients think and feel about themselves as well as how they are regarded by others (Hacking, 2013).

Classifications and their consequences, as Bowker and Star (1999) suggest, facilitate connections between individuals and their bodies as well as wider systems of governance, regulation and new forms of knowledge. Foucault urges us to think of these connections in terms of 'two poles of development linked together by a whole cluster of intermediary relations' (Foucault in Hacking, 1995: 215). One pole centres on the individual as a speaking, working, procreating entity – what Foucault calls an 'anatomo-politics of the human body'. The second pole focuses on how this body serves as the 'basis of the biological processes: propagation, births, and mortality, the level of health, life expectancy and longevity' (Hacking, 1995: 215). Foucault calls this polarity a 'biopolitics', a concept that has been critical for subsequent social scientific work on the interplay between bodies at individual and population levels (Flower and Heath, 1993; Agamben, 1998; Hardt and Negri, 2000; Esposito, 2008). Biopolitics is less concerned with bodies as sites of lived experience or objects of discipline, and more with aggregates of bodies as the site for the application of metrics that enable measurement, monitoring and governance, organized through the disciplines of statistics, demography, epidemiology and genetics. Put another way, biopolitics relates to the instruments for regulation and control, rather than discipline and supervision (Lemke, 2011).

The 'engines of discovery' that constitute biopolitical subjects transform individual bodies into new categories: 'population objects' (Ruppert, 2011). Evelyn Ruppert's work shows how identification and classificatory practices, such as censuses, population registers, disease and health registries, and identification cards, have become critical for monitoring the transactions, communications and movements of individuals under the imperatives of combating terrorism, fraud, illegal migration, epidemic threats and so on. While the changing nature of population metrics and scale and reach of population databases is generating new methodological, theoretical and analytic challenges for the social sciences, we need to be cautious not to treat such technologies of 'legibility' (Scott, 1998) as straightforwardly reflecting state power, or of governmental intention or capacity to intervene.

The preceding sections work to present an understanding of the body as something less defined by a set of intrinsic or essential attributes than by the sets of arrangements within which we as embodied subjects connect to the world. In what follows, we crystallize the kinds of complementary insights these approaches offer through a case study on the rise of neuroscientific models of addiction. Although the brain, the central focus of this section, sits ambiguously within the mind–body dyad, it has become an increasingly central means through which we 'know' ourselves, as well as being part of the embodied conditions through which we experience and relate to the world around us.

Conceptualizing addiction

Although the concept of addiction has been with us for several hundred years, it continues to be the source of considerable discussion and debate: 'Is addiction a disease or a learnt behaviour? Is it a property of drugs or of individuals? Are different addictions the expression of one overarching disorder or are they distinct pathologies?' (Keane, 1999: 64). As these questions suggest, addiction has always resisted definitive attempts at classification. However, instead of treating it as merely the *object* of classification, we might be better served by treating it as the *product*. Considered from this standpoint, the addicted subject is materially constituted through 'a multiplicity of organisms, forces, energies, materials, desire, thoughts, etc.' (Foucault, 1980: 97). It is this material constitution of the 'addict' that we detail below, focusing on the modes of classification that produce her and the kinds of disciplining it gives rise to via new forms of intervention, before turning to the ways it organizes the embodied experience of addiction.

There are currently two dominant models for conceptualizing and classifying addiction: the 'mental disorder' model and the 'brain disease' model (Fraser et al., 2014). The 'mental disorder' model of addiction is outlined in the DSM and its inclusion establishes 'substance use disorders' as a pathological condition requiring therapeutic intervention. To quote Suzanne Fraser and colleagues (2014: 34), 'the manual enacts addiction as a condition more like depression or schizophrenia and less like other things, such as an everyday bad habit, a sin, a lifestyle or a physical disease such as an allergy'. As Robin Room observes:

> the addiction concept is... a term used to describe what is perceived and defined as a mystery: the mystery of the drinker or drug user continuing to use despite what is seen as the harm – such as casualties, damage to health, and failures of work and family roles – resulting from use.
>
> (Room, 2003: 225)

However, since the 1990s, neuroscience has become an increasingly authoritative source of knowledge about addiction (Keane, 1999; Rose, 2003; Courtwright, 2010; Vrecko, 2010; Netherland, 2011; Fraser et al., 2014; Raikhel, 2015). In categorizing these developments, Nikolas Rose (2003: 407) notes that addiction is increasingly seen not as a 'disease of the will' but a 'disease of the brain'. In other words, 'the brain' has increasingly supplemented both 'the mind' and 'the body' as a means of conceptualizing addiction – although, as we will see below, it instantiates a particular view of both.

The neuroscience of addiction and the 'hijacked' brain

Neuroscientific accounts of addiction emphasize the ways in which chronic drug use creates changes in the brain that impair users' voluntary control over their behaviour (Carter et al., 2012). In this framing, drugs – and other pleasurable activities such as gambling, food, sex and so on – can 'hijack' the brain mechanisms involved in seeking natural reinforcement (see Keane, 1999; Campbell, 2010; Vrecko, 2010; Netherland, 2011; Fraser et al., 2014; Raikhel, 2015). These pathological changes are manifested in a behavioural disorder characterized by uncontrollable, compulsive drug craving that persists in the face of negative social and health consequences.

The National Institute on Drug Abuse (NIDA) in the USA has been a key advocate of the view that persistent use of drugs leads to long-term changes in the structure and function of the brain, with addiction defined as a 'chronic, relapsing brain disease' (Courtwright, 2010: 137). Nevertheless, this characterization is largely a reframing of a series of hypotheses posited from the 1920s, which similarly held that drug addictions were connected by a common pathological action on the nervous system, itself permanently altered by drug use (Courtwright, 2010; Campbell, 2010). Although these models share various characteristics, as Eugene Raikhel (2015) points out, they invoke distinct loci and mechanisms for addiction, privileging different forms of intervention, disciplinary techniques and lines of scientific inquiry.

Central to the rise of the brain-disease model of addiction was the emergence of neuro-imaging technologies that enabled scientists to visualize the effects of addiction on the brain (Keane, 1999; Dumit, 2004; Campbell, 2010; Netherland, 2011;

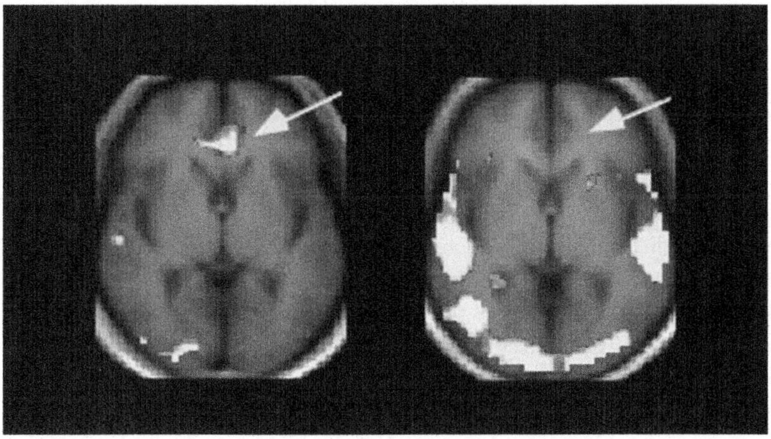

FIGURE 7.1 Functional magnetic resonance images of the brain of a 'cocaine-addicted' patient (left) and a healthy volunteer (right) (Source: reproduced from Fowler et al., 2007).

Fraser et al., 2014). For example, in an article titled 'Imaging the addicted human brain', Fowler et al. (2007: 4) state: 'scientific advances of the last quarter century have established that drug addiction is a chronic brain disease. Key evidence for this view consists of images of people's brains taken during or following drug exposures.' Providing an overview of various brain imaging techniques, the article features numerous images of the brains of 'addicted' patients contrasted with those of 'normal' people (see Figure 7.1).

Here we clearly see the 'making up' of the 'addict' as a specific kind of person (Hacking, 2006) through a sociocultural apparatus that presents itself in technical garb. As Joseph Dumit (2004) observes, although brain imaging technologies presume to portray certain *kinds* of brains that are, in turn, presumed to belong to certain *kinds* of person, these ways of thinking about the brain have a very particular social history. For example, Fraser et al. (2014) point out that although NIDA scientists invoke an organic vision of addiction, one in which it is produced as a physiological as opposed to psychological phenomenon, scientists quickly shift from terms like 'improper inhibitory control' to 'aberrant behaviour' (see also Keane and Hamill, 2010; Netherland, 2011). Thus, despite the ways that such formulations equate the 'diseased addicted brain' with the 'diseased heart', the brain is also *not* like the heart but is read as equivalent to the self: 'a disordered brain equals a disordered self and a disordered life' (Fraser et al., 2014: 55).

Likewise, Dumit notes that PET scans used to image the heart are fundamentally different from brain images of mind and personhood. This is because the former can be calibrated directly with their referent: the heart can be looked at surgically and we can learn exactly what signals correspond with different tissue states. Images of the 'addicted brain' or the 'schizophrenic' or 'depressed' one cannot be verified in the same way. However, despite the cultural and visual logics 'by which these images persuade viewers to equate person with brain, brain with scan, and scan with diagnosis' (Dumit, 2004: 6), they are presented as both self-evident and indisputable.

Treating the addicted brain, training the addict

The rise of neuroscientific research has served to transform the ways we understand and respond to addiction – both collectively and individually – providing new contours to governance and shaping new kinds of subjects (Netherland, 2011). As Rose (2003: 414) observes, 'these processes were not merely processes of discovery, but of intervention – the neurochemical brain becomes known in the very same process that invents interventions to manipulate its functioning – that is to say, therapeutic drugs'. As the brain-disease model has grown more influential, pharmaceutical technologies targeting the biochemical processes of the brain have been developed as potential treatments, including naltrexone, which is understood to reduce sensations of craving, and buprenorphine, a synthetic opioid that works by blocking the pleasurable effects of other opioids (Rose, 2003; Netherland, 2011; Raikhel, 2015). Although such psycho-pharmaceutical treatments are not widely available, it's likely that they will increasingly supplement the prevailing disciplinary techniques that produce the addict-in-recovery, namely 12-step programmes.

Neuroscientists insist that such approaches and the new responses to addiction they engender will usher in a new era in which addiction is dealt with in medical as opposed to crimino-legal settings. However, 'neurochemical explanations of addiction continue to reflect and reproduce the pathological figure of the addict whose life has been destroyed by the inherently destructive power of drugs' (Keane and Hamill, 2010: 57–58; see also Fraser et al., 2014). According to Nancy Campbell (2010), although constructs such as 'compulsion', 'disruption' and 'disinhibition' are presented as novel outcomes of neuroscientific knowledge, they owe a substantial debt to older configurations of addiction as a moral weakness or disease of the will. Indeed, the brain-disease model 'would never have taken hold had it not converged with recovery discourse and become effective at organizing meanings in the popular realm' (Campbell, 2010: 93).

Campbell (2010) illustrates the synergy between the brain-disease model of addiction and earlier ideological codes by reference to an episode of the *Oprah Winfrey Show* featuring the neuroscientist Anna Rose Childress and her patient, William, who was being treated for cocaine addiction. As a neuroscientist, Childress saw herself as engaged in countering the stigma attached to addiction, but audience members and Oprah herself kept shifting conversation from the neurophysiology of relapse to the moral imperative not to use. Campbell points out that the audience's response reveals just how little public perceptions about addiction as a matter of personal responsibility and choice have shifted with the rise of neuroscience. After all, while neuro-scientific constructions of relapse as beyond conscious control differ from popular notions of morality, they nevertheless raise questions of individual variation: why can some people stop but not others?

Experiencing the addicted brain

As older models of addiction have come to be supplemented (if not entirely supplanted) by the brain-disease model, we have seen the rise of what Rose (2003) terms 'neurochemical selves'. In his words, 'we can see a shift in the kinds of persons upon which government will act – the birth, that is to say, of genetic and neurochemical selfhood' (Rose, 2003: 408). Julie Netherland's (2011) research with 37 US patients being treated for addiction with buprenorphine for opiate dependence provides one such illustration of the ways in which subjectivities are shaped by 'folk neurology'. Participants frequently emphasized the effectiveness of buprenorphine in blocking the pleasurable effects of drugs, with 'Mr S' observing: 'Bup[renorphine] is like a condom on the brain. You know, you don't *feel* the heroin' (Netherland, 2011: 161, emphasis added). However, this non-feeling was itself commonly experienced as a *feeling*. As Netherland (2011: 162) observes, 'treatment went beyond restrictive control of cravings to proscriptive achievement of a very particular kind of personhood, of being "extra normal"'.

However, participants also insisted that the drug alone could not produce 'recovery'; for that, will power was required, along with changes in their social circumstances that might facilitate such change (help with employment, housing, mental health, and so on). Thus, 'buprenorphine blocked the cravings, but sheer determination stopped the drug use' (Netherland, 2011: 170). Such accounts illustrate the ways in which participants were unwilling to fully cede control of their brains and bodies to medicine, leading to a blended view of addiction: a disease in one instance, a problem of will power and character in another. As these narratives demonstrate, the idea of addiction as a defect in the brain increased rather than diminished a sense of personal responsibility, with the quest to be 'normal' encompassing 'a way of life characterized by autonomous, responsible citizenship often achieved through will power and medication' (Netherland, 2011: 172). Thus, we clearly see the ways in which the embodied experience of addiction is fundamentally informed by technologies that classify 'the addicted brain' and aim to treat it, but are nevertheless irreducible to such.

Conclusion

The body has without doubt generated a vast array of scholarship and stands as a critical site for the generation of concepts: concepts that manifest ways of thinking on and with the body. The various tensions revealed in conceptual work on the body crystallize the inseparability of subject–object relations and the futility of prioritizing one over the other – which can only lead us down barren cul-de-sacs that produce neither chickens nor eggs, despite endlessly debating both. This inseparability has been taken up in various ways by the three approaches we have detailed. All attempt to destabilize subject–object distinctions in various ways: by showing how such distinctions are grounded in the experience of the body; by showing how ways of working with the body manifest it as the nexus of the individual and the social; and by showing how systems of classification actively 'make up' people with particular kinds of bodies.

In all cases, we are shown the various ways in which bodies become important, under what circumstances and for whom. Taking these three framings together, it is also clear that the very tensions that mark out the subject–object distinctions that scholarship on the body depends upon have been shown to be enormously productive for social science scholarship. These tensions constitute *our* 'engines of discovery' – ones that provide us not only with a rich conceptual landscape for articulating the body, but the methodological approaches that underpin them. Thus, in starting with the body and moving outwards from its boundaries, as we have done, we become aware of the social and cultural worlds within which it finds its particular moorings and modes of understanding.

Notes

1 We emphasize 'productivity' here in the sense that the body becomes a site of knowledge production – a potent means of generating knowledge across a wide range of disciplines, something that has been as central to the work of Michel Foucault (1975, 1978) and also Judith Butler (1993), Elizabeth Grosz (1994) and Bruno Latour (1999), as it has in the biosciences. In reflecting on the body we are, therefore, also reflecting on the processes of knowledge production.

2 The volume of readers and compendiums on the body is far too vast for us to list here; but we would recommend Shilling (1993), Lock and Farquhar (2007) and Moore and Casper (2014) as useful introductions.

3 For further thinking on feminism and the body, see Davis (1997), Price and Shildrick (1999) and Schiebinger (2000).

4 We note here that others have offered related categorizations of ways to understand the body. In addition to Scheper-Hughes and Lock's three bodies, we can also refer to O'Neill's five bodies (2004) and Mol's 'body multiple' (2003). However, for us, the relevant question is not one of number. While our scheme also works with a 'three bodies' framing, we would like to emphasize some differences. We do not intend the organization of this chapter to work as an overarching description or categorization of scholarship in this area, but as a heuristic – a device for highlighting the ways in which tensions or dualisms have produced conceptual ways of working with the body. In doing so, we start with the individual experience and work outwards to issues of governmentality in order to emphasize the connections rather than the distinctions between approaches.

5 Karen Barad (2007), for instance, has shown how these issues were taken up in quantum mechanics. According to Barad, for Niels Bohr, in his Nobel Prize-winning work in physics, the problem to be resolved was that humans were both part of measuring systems as well as part of that being measured and so were, at one and the same time, both inside and outside the physical world.

6 In *Primate Visions*, Donna Haraway (1989: 139) defines the cyborg as an entity in which 'two kinds of boundary are simultaneously problematic... a figure born of the interface of automation and autonomy'.

7 In her writings on cyborgs, Haraway talks about the techno-scientific relations of production in an adaptation of and contemporary reworking of Marx (see Chapter 4 for further discussion). Haraway has always underlined her engagement with the work of Marx but has done so in the context of an ongoing dialogue with feminism and the social scientific production of knowledge.

8 In his account of habitus, while Bourdieu gestures in the direction of the knowing subject (i.e., the autonomous agent), he has little to say about it.
9 Although Foucault was interested in broader historical shifts in modes of objectification of the body, in his later work (see Foucault, 1993), he refuted the idea of a straightforward transition from technologies of domination to technologies of the self, noting that the scholar 'has to take into account the points where the technologies of domination of individuals over one another have recourse to processes by which the individual acts upon himself. And conversely, he has to take into account the points where the techniques of the self are integrated into structures of coercion and domination' (p. 203).
10 In *Disciplining Foucault* (1991), Jana Sawicki shows how Foucault's analysis of categorization and representation can be extended to open up feminist controversies on identity, difference and the place of the 'mother' in their formations.
11 For a similar approach, see Latour (1987) on the production of scientific facts.

References

Agamben, G. (1998) *Homo Sacer: Sovereign Power and Bare Life*. Stanford, CA: Stanford University Press.

Barad, K. (2007) *Meeting the University Half-Way: Quantum Physics and the Entanglement of Matter and Meaning*. Durham, NC: Duke University Press.

Bourdieu, P. (1996) Vilhelm Aubert Memorial Lecture: *Physical Space, Social Space and Habitus*. Department of Sociology: University of Oslo & Institute for Social Research.

Bowker, G. and Star, S.L. (1999) *Sorting Things Out: Classification and its Consequences*. Cambridge, MA: MIT Press.

Butler, J. (1993) *Bodies that Matter: On the Discursive Limits of Sex*. London: Routledge.

Campbell, N. (2010) Toward a critical neuroscience of 'addiction'. *BioSocieties*, 5(1): 89–104.

Carter, A., Hall, W. and Illes, J. (eds.) (2012) *Addiction Neuroethics: The Ethics of Addiction Neuroscience Research and Treatment*. London: Academic Press.

Casper, M. (1995) Fetal cyborgs and technomoms on the reproductive frontier: which way to the carnival? In C. Hables Gray (ed.), *The Cyborg Handbook*, New York: Routledge, 183–202.

Courtwright, D.T. (2010) The NIDA brain disease paradigm: history, resistance and spinoffs. *BioSocieties*, 5(1): 137–147.

Csordas, T. (1994) *Embodiment and Experience: The Existential Ground of Culture and Self*. Cambridge: Cambridge University Press.

Davis, K. (1997) *Embodied Practices: Feminist Perspectives on the Body*. London: Sage.

Davis Floyd, R. (1994) The technocratic body: American childbirth as cultural expression. *Social Science and Medicine*, 38: 1125–1140.

DelVecchio Good, M., Brodwin, P.E., Good, B.J. and Kleinman, A. (eds.) (1994) *Pain as Human Experience: An Anthropological Perspective*. Berkeley, CA: University of California Press.

Douglas, M. (1966) *Purity and Danger*. London: Routledge and Kegan Paul.

Douglas, M. (1973) *Natural Symbols*. Harmondsworth: Penguin.

Dreyfus, H. and Rabinow, P. (1983) *Michel Foucault: Beyond Structuralism and Hermenutics*. Chicago, IL: University of Chicago Press.

Dumit, J. (1995) Brain-mind machines and American technological dream marketing: towards an ethnography of cyborg envy. In C. Hables Gray (ed.), *The Cyborg Handbook*, New York: Routledge, 347–362.

Dumit, J. (2004) *Picturing Personhood: Brain Scans and Biomedical Identity*. Durham, NC: Duke University Press.
Esposito, R. (2008) *Bíos: Biopolitics and Philosophy*. Minneapolis, MN: University of Minnesota Press.
Flower, M. and Heath, D. (1993) Micro-anatomo politics: mapping the human genome project. *Culture, Medicine and Psychiatry*, 17: 27–41.
Foucault, M. (1970) *The Order of Things: An Archaeology of the Human Sciences*. New York: Random House.
Foucault, M. (1975) *Discipline and Punish: The Birth of the Prison*. London: Penguin.
Foucault, M. (1978) *The History of Sexuality, Volume 1: An Introduction*. New York: Random House.
Foucault, M. (1980) *Power and Knowledge: Selected Interviews and Other Writings, 1972–1977*. Translated by C. Gordon. New York: Pantheon.
Foucault, M. (1993) About the beginning of the hermeneutics of the self: two lectures at Dartmouth. *Political Theory*, 21(2): 198–277.
Fowler, J.S., Volkow, N.D., Kassed, C.A. and Chang, L. (2007) Imaging the addicted human brain. *Addiction Science and Clinical Practice*, 3(2): 4–16.
Fraser, S., Moore, D. and Keane, H. (2014) *Habits: Remaking Addiction*. London: Palgrave Macmillan.
Goffman, E. (1961) *Asylums: Essays on the Social Situation of Mental Patients and Other Inmates*. New York: Anchor Books.
Grosz, E. (1994) *Volatile Bodies: Toward a Corporeal Feminism*. Bloomington, IN: Indiana University Press.
Hables Gray, C. (2002) *Cyborg Citizen*. New York: Routledge.
Hacking, I. (1995) *Rewriting the Soul: Multiple Personality and the Sciences of Memory*. Princeton, NJ: Princeton University Press.
Hacking, I. (2000) *The Social Construction of What?* Harvard, MA: Harvard University Press.
Hacking, I. (2006) Making up people. *London Review of Books*, 28(16): 23–26.
Hacking, I. (2013) Lost in the forest. *London Review of Books*, 35(15): 7–8.
Haraway, D. (1989) *Primate Visions: Gender, Race, and Nature in the World of Modern Science*. New York: Routledge.
Haraway, D. (1991) *Simians, Cyborgs and Women: The Reinvention of Nature*. New York: Routledge.
Hardt, M. and Negri, A. (2000) *Empire*. Boston, MA: Harvard University Press.
Hobbes, T. (2012 [1651]) *Leviathan*. Edited by N. Malcom. Oxford: Oxford University Press.
Jackson, J. (1994) Chronic pain and the tension between the body as subject and object. In T. Csordas (ed.), *Embodiment and Experience: The Existential Ground of Culture and Self*. Cambridge: Cambridge University Press, 201–228.
Keane, H. (1999) Adventures of the addicted brain. *Australian Feminist Studies*, 14(29): 63–76.
Keane, H. and Hamill, K. (2010) Variations in addiction: the molecular and the molar in neuroscience and pain medicine. *BioSocieties*, 5(1): 52–69.
Latour, B. (1987) *Science in Action: How to Follow Scientists and Engineers through Society*. Cambridge MA: Harvard University Press.
Latour, B. (1999) *Pandora's Hope: Essays on the Reality of Science Studies*. Chicago, IL: Chicago University Press.
Latour, B. (2004) How to talk about the body? The normative dimension of science studies. *Body and Society*, 10(2–3): 205–229.
Leder, D. (1990) *The Absent Body*. Chicago, IL: University of Chicago Press.
Lemke, T. (2011) *Bio-Politics: An Advanced Introduction*. New York: New York University Press.
Lock, M. and Farquhar, J. (eds.) (2007) *Beyond the Body Proper: Reading the Anthropology of Material Life*. Durham, NC: Duke University Press.
Martin, E. (1987) *The Woman in the Body*. Milton Keynes: Open University Press.

Mauss, M. (1992 [1934]) The techniques of the body. In J. Crary and S. Kwinter (eds.), *Incorporations*. New York: Zone, 455–477.
Merleau-Ponty, M. (1962) *The Phenomenology of Perception*. Translated by J. Wild and J.M. Edie. Evanston, IL: Northwestern University Press.
Merleau-Ponty, M. (1964) *Signs*. Evanston, IL: Northwestern University Press.
Miller, J. (2000) *The Body in Question*. London: Pimlico.
Mol, A. (2003) *The Body Multiple: Ontology in Medical Practice*. Durham, NC: Duke University Press.
Moore, L.J. and Casper, M. (2014) *The Body: Social and Cultural Dissections*. London: Routledge.
Navarro, Z. (2006) In search of cultural interpretation of power. *IDS Bulletin*, 37(6): 11–22.
Netherland, J. (2011) 'We haven't sliced open anyone's brain yet': neuroscience, embodiment and the governance of addiction. In M. Pickersgill and I. Van Keulen (eds.), *Sociological Reflections on the Neurosciences*, 13: 153–177.
O'Neill, J. (2004) *Five Bodies: Re-figuring Relationships*. London: Sage.
Price, J. and Shildrick, M. (1999) *Feminist Theory and the Body: A Reader*. Edinburgh: Edinburgh University Press.
Porter, R. (2003) *Flesh in the Age of Reason*. London: Allen Lane.
Raikhel, E. (2015) From the brain disease model to ecologies of addiction. In L. Kirmayer, R. Lemelson and C. Cummings (eds.), *Revisioning Psychiatry: Cultural Phenomenology, Critical Neuroscience, and Global Mental Health*. Cambridge: Cambridge University Press.
Regier, D.A., Kuhl, E.A. and Kupfer, D.J. (2013) The DSM-5: classification and criteria changes. *World Psychiatry*, 12(2): 92–98.
Room, R. (2003) The cultural framing of addiction. *Janus Head*, 6(2): 221–234.
Rose, N. (2003) The neurochemical self and its anomalies. In R.V. Erickson and A. Doyle (eds.), *Risk and Morality*. Toronto: University of Toronto Press, 407–437.
Ruppert, E. (2011) Population objects: interpassive subjects. *Sociology*, 45(2): 218–233.
Sawday, J. (1995) *The Body Emblazoned*. London: Routledge.
Sawicki, J. (1991) *Disciplining Foucault: Gender, Power, and the Body*. London: Routledge.
Scarry, E. (1985) *The Body in Pain*. Oxford: Oxford University Press.
Scheper-Hughes, N. and Lock, M.M. (1987) The mindful body: a prolegomenon to future work in medical anthropology. *Medical Anthropology Quarterly*, 1(1): 6–41.
Schiebinger, L. (2000) *Feminism and the Body*. Oxford: Oxford University Press.
Schutz, A. (1971) On multiple realities. In *Collected Papers, Vol. 1: The Problem of Social Reality*. The Hague: Martinus Nijhoff, 207–259.
Scott, J.C. (1998) *Seeing Like a State: How Certain Schemes to Improve the Human Condition Have Failed*. New Haven, CT: Yale University Press.
Shilling, C. (1993) *The Body and Social Theory*. London: Sage.
Vrecko, S. (2010) Birth of a brain disease: science, the state and addiction neuropolitics. *History of the Human Sciences*, 23(4): 52–67.
Young, K. (1997) *Presence in the Flesh: the Body in Medicine*. Cambridge: Harvard University Press.

CONCLUSION

In February 2015, British Members of Parliament approved a proposed change in law that would enable the conception of 'three-person babies'. This legislative amendment would allow UK fertility clinics to carry out mitochondrial donation, an IVF technique that involves biological material from three people. In essence, the mitochondrial DNA of a woman with mitochondrial disease would be swapped with that of an anonymous female donor. Thus, 99.8 per cent of genetic material would come from the mother and father and 0.2 per cent from the mitochondrial donor (Devlin, 2015).

In the UK, the public face of the procedure was Sharon Bernardi, a Sunderland woman who lost seven children to Leigh's Disease (Dicker, 2012). In an open letter published in *The Mirror* in 2013 she wrote:

> This is not about being selfish… It is not about creating babies with a certain type of hair or certain colour of eyes. It is about giving parents the option of trying to create a healthy baby. A baby that lives and grows up. It's about trying to give a child a future.
>
> (Bernardi, 2013)

As Bernardi's comments suggest, the procedure itself is highly controversial, with many worried that it will pave the way for 'designer babies' (Clark, 2013; Gallagher, 2015).[1] While advocates point out that the goal is to save lives, not 'manufacture' improved offspring, critics argue that the difference between 'correctionist' and 'selectionist' eugenics is a matter of degree (Clark, 2013). Others worry about what it would mean to have three biological parents. For some, a three-person baby so radically undermines the genetic basis of kinship, offspring could have 'no true genetic parents'; others wonder what claims the 'second mother' (i.e., the mitochondrial donor) might be able to make – if any – over the resultant offspring (Clark, 2013).

In light of these concerns, intensive discussion has centred on what role mitochondrial versus nuclear genes play in determining personal identity. Some opponents also worry about the social consequences if such technologies are only available to certain segments of the population (i.e., the wealthy) and their potential to create new forms of class distinction – 'Gattaca-style eugenics' as it is frequently labelled, referencing the 1997 science-fiction film set in a not-too-distant future where society is divided into genetically engineered 'valids' and everybody else ('invalids'). For such critics, cures, if introduced at all, would need to be freely available to everybody (Clark, 2013).

The debate generated by 'three-person babies' demonstrates the ongoing salience of the core concepts we have explored in this book as they mediate the intersections between medicine, technology and society and help us to make sense of them. First and foremost, it provides insights into how notions of relatedness are worked out (Chapter 5). Despite the clear emphasis on the biogenetic basis of kinship in the debate, the questions it raises reveal the ways in which nature has been destabilized as a fixed referent. This becomes especially evident in concerns that three-person babies would entirely undermine the genetic basis of kinship. The notion of the gift and the relations of exchange it establishes (Chapter 6) provides insight into these concerns, especially questions about what obligations the act of mitochondrial donation might incur for the recipient. It also makes sense of the insistence that donors remain anonymous – which was a key condition for approving the change in law. We might also consider the abundance of production metaphors in the debate – 'manufactured' children and so on – and the ways they speak to concerns about the enmeshment of reproduction with production as a wider social form (Chapter 4). Questions about the consequences of such technologies on relationships – between parents and children, between classes – also make visible the social and cultural conditions within which these technologies are anticipated to work (Chapters 1 and 2).

Attempts to disentangle the biological and social aspects of personhood (does identity spring from nuclear genes? Does it spring from our upbringing?) also speak to the ongoing pervasiveness of efforts to establish the origins and destinies – and causes and consequences – of these biotechnical developments (Chapter 3). Finally, the debate is unquestionably about the status and role of the body, not only as a simultaneous object and subject, but the ways in which it functions as a worksite – one in which we are, in addition, its engineer and architect (Chapter 7). The changing character of human embodiment, in particular the ways technology works upon the body's affordances to transform its shape, functions and prospects, also enables us to move out to wider concerns about the 'cyborgification' of selves and the ways in which multiple actors are working to create new possibilities for us as a species. These concerns, and the hopes and anxieties they invoke, are not new; they have been with us since Marx, and continue to have relevance.

Importantly, while the concepts we have examined help us to make sense of the cluster of issues bound up with three-person babies (as but one example), they also throw into relief the persistence of dualistic thinking – nature/culture and individual/society splits – and their continued influence over the production of knowledge. As we have seen, these dichotomies structured thinking around all the concepts to varying degrees, even as empirical work repeatedly troubled them. Much of this scholarship revealed attempts to hive off the biological and cultural as unsustainable – whether it is worked through the lens of 'culture', 'magic', 'kinship' or 'the body'. Likewise, efforts to settle the relationship between society and the individual (via concepts such as 'society', 'production', 'exchange' and 'the body') prove to be provisional and constantly refigured due to the impossibility of delineating the two, once and for all. This work suggested that relations between individuals and society are continually made and remade through this dichotomy, which is simultaneously restrictive and enabling.

Rather than providing us with a set of problems to be resolved or challenged in a one-sided fashion, the dualisms that intimately underpin work across the sciences (social and natural) provide instead a fertile ground for examination and exploration, indeed a productive ground, one in which conceptual developments thrive. Interestingly, this is not just about polemical critique and opposition, but also the potential for mutual elaboration. Thus, if biomedicine continues to be 'caught in the clutches of the Cartesian dichotomy', these dichotomies have also been 'good to think' with (Scheper-Hughes and Lock, 1987: 30). Indeed, it is by attending to developments in science, medicine and technology that we continue to refine the conceptual ground that has become a hallmark of anthropology and sociology.

In working with concepts, our goal has not been to invoke them as a way of producing neat, pre-packaged explanations for phenomena or, indeed, as prescriptions for doing research. As Bruno Latour notes, when sociologists and anthropologists pronounce the words 'society', 'culture' and so on:

> they often jump straight ahead to connect vast arrays of life and history, to mobilize gigantic forces, to detect dramatic patterns emerging out of confusing interactions, to see everywhere in the cases at hand yet more examples of well-known types, to reveal behind the scenes some dark powers pulling the strings.
>
> (Latour, 2005: 22)

Instead, our concern has been to explore their enduring features, the ways they frame our understanding of phenomena (for better, but also for worse), and their uses both inside and outside the social sciences.

By examining the uses to which these concepts can be and have been put – in terms of their topography, their analytical potentials and constraints, as well as the controversies they give rise to – we have shown how they open up scientific, medical and technical practice to various modes of examination and explication. In doing so, we hope that we have offered our readers valuable avenues of exploration, methodologically and theoretically, and a set of signposts within which they can position their own methodological interests and topics of concern.

Note

1 These concerns are far from new and have repeatedly been raised in the context of developments in a variety of reproductive and genetic technologies (see Chapter 4).

References

Bernardi, S. (2013) Three-parent babies: mum who lost seven children to rare genetic disease backs move. *The Mirror*. Available at: www.mirror.co.uk/news/real-life-stories/three-parent-babies-mum-who-lost-2007652.

Clark, L. (2013) In depth: three-person IVF is about saving lives, not a slippery slope to eugenics. *Wired*. Available at: www.wired.co.uk/news/archive/2013-06/28/mitochondria-transfer-ruling.

Devlin, H. (2015) Britain's House of Lords approves conception of three-person babies. *The Guardian*. Available at: www.theguardian.com/politics/2015/feb/24/uk-house-of-lords-approves-conception-of-three-person-babies.

Dicker, R. (2012) Sharon Bernardi loses 7 children to Leigh's Disease – but hopes for cure. *Huffington Post*. Available at: www.huffingtonpost.com/2012/09/20/sharon-bernardi_n_1900248.html.

Gallagher, J. (2015) MPs say yes to three-person babies. *BBC News*. Available at: www.bbc.com/news/health-31069173.

Latour, B. (2005) *Reassembling the Social: An Introduction to Actor-Network-Theory*. Oxford: Oxford University Press.

Scheper-Hughes, N. and Lock, M.M. (1987) The mindful body: a prolegomenon to future work in medical anthropology. *Medical Anthropology Quarterly*, 1(1): 6–41.

INDEX

Walki
Tees

by
Keith Watson

DALESMAN BOOKS
1978

75p.

THE DALESMAN PUBLISHING COMPANY LTD.,
CLAPHAM (Via Lancaster), NORTH YORKSHIRE

First Published 1978

ISBN: O 85206 485 3

Printed in Great Britain by
GEO. TODD & SON,
Marlborough Street, Whitehaven

CONTENTS

Cover illustration of Romaldkirk by Alec Wright.

Drawing of the Market Cross, Barnard Castle, and maps by Christopher J. Coulthard.

THE COUNTRY CODE

Guard against all Risk of Fire

Fasten all Gates

Keep Dogs under Proper Control

Keep to the Paths across Farm Land

Avoid Damaging Fences, Hedges and Walls

Leave No Litter

Safeguard Water Supplies

Protect Wild Life, Wild Plants and Trees

Go Carefully on Country Roads

Respect the Life of the Countryside

FOREWORD

TEESDALE, with its grand peat-brown river, green and flower-scattered pastures, heather-clad fells, is not only beautiful but also relatively undiscovered — one of the last unspoiled places in the country. Other Pennine and Cumbrian dales have been all but overwhelmed by the annual flood of tourists, but Teesdale remains almost unmarked, with a welcome for discerning visitors which is still friendly, spontaneous and infinitely rewarding.

It is a significant part of my work to help ensure that this happy balance is maintained — visitors should come on dalesfolks' terms, so that both townsman and countryman may benefit. This book is intended to help maintain the balance: it will lead the active visitor by paths which are safe and trouble-free rights of way to a full enjoyment of many of Teesdale's hidden delights.

In return, we hope for sensible and considerate behaviour from our visitors — know and understand the Country Code and you will not go far wrong. Bear in mind also that the same fellsides and pastures which offer recreation to the townsman must provide a living for the countryman, and that this living is very much the concern of us all: efficient farming raises our standard of living and lowers our import bill, and the visitor can readily influence this equation for better or worse.

Most of the walks in this book are through the woodlands and meadows of the Tees and its tributaries, and can be tackled by anyone reasonably fit, well shod and sensibly clad. Fell walks in the upper dale are in a different world, though, where the combination of climate, elevation and aspect can threaten even the most experienced and the best prepared. Equip yourself for safety and comfort on the fells, add the Mountain Code to the Country Code for guidance, and keep a weather eye open.

Good walking!

SIMON HODGSON,
Durham Countryside Warden.

INTRODUCTION

THE PRIMARY PURPOSE of this book is two fold, firstly to provide a much needed and up-to-date volume of walks of Teesdale, and secondly to describe walks of varied distances which are suitable for the walker-motorist, youth hosteller and experienced walker. I have selected 15 walks and for each there is a sketch map, which should be used for reference only, and recommend that it is essential always to carry an Ordnance Survey map of the area, details of which are included separately under each walk. Thirteen walks are circular and suitable for the motorist, two walks are non-circular and ideal for the youth hosteller, while certain adjoining routes can provide walks for the experienced walker. The paths described are all public rights of way.

Details of public transport have been included where applicable for those walkers without their own transport. However, care must be taken when planning walks if public transport is used, as timetables are subject to alteration or cancellation, particularly when more and more rural public transport is being withdrawn. The Durham County Timetable (includes United Automobile Services Ltd., G.N.E. Motor Services and Teesdale Coach Services which serve Teesdale) is a valuable guide.

The walks vary in length from 2 to 17 miles and are suitable for all walkers to enjoy, providing they are adequately equipped for such walks. Therefore, I recommend that everyone, especially the inexperienced walker, equip himself by wearing strong footwear, preferably walking boots which support the ankles and help to prevent sprains and blisters. Thick wool socks, anorak, warm clothing including a sweater, and waterproofs, such as a cagoule, should be worn. A rucksack can be useful to carry the following items — waterproofs; extra warm clothing; sufficient food; plastic bag for rubbish; thermos flask; compass; an Ordnance Survey map of the area; torch; whistle; emergency rations (preferably containing energy and warmth-producing food); and first aid equipment.

I must stress and emphasise that great care must be taken when attempting walks in the Middleton area, especially the Langdon Beck — High Cup Nick walk, where a walker died and two others suffered from exposure some years ago. In addition, many mild cases of exposure are frequent in this area. It is essential that walkers plan their routes carefully, and should take into consideration the terrain of the area, allowance of time, notification of route to a responsible person and the weather conditions, where often rain, mist and wind can cause cold and exhaustion resulting in possible exposure. In the case of emergency, the Upper Teesdale/Weardale Fell Rescue Association cover the area and are available through the 999 Mountain Rescue Emergency calls or by the Police — I hope you never have the need to call out the Association.

Each walk includes historical and natural information to stimulate the walkers' interest and intense research has been undertaken to record the facts accurately. The text has been divided into three parts —

1. Walks around Barnard Castle.
2. Walks around Middleton-in-Teesdale.
3. Hostel to Hostel.

Since the author walked the following routes, it is inevitable that certain changes have occurred in the Teesdale countryside. It is not always possible to keep up to date and I apologise for any alterations.

Finally, please remember the safety code and observe the County Code and, most of all, enjoy your walks and visits to Teesdale.

KEITH WATSON,
Norton,
Cleveland.

TEESDALE

TEESDALE described in this text relates to the extensive area of country between Barnard Castle and Middleton-in-Teesdale. Upstream from High Force and including Cauldron Snout is known as Upper Teesdale, which is renowned for its wild grandeur and romantic scenery. On 1st April, 1974, Teesdale was officially recognised as a District Council, due to Local Government reform. The District comprises the former Barnard Castle Urban, Barnard Castle Rural and Startforth Rural Councils which ceased to exist —the latter Council was located in North Yorkshire. Hence, Yorkshire was deprived of the attractive villages of Bowes, Cotherstone, Romaldkirk, Mickleton and Holwick; and well known landmarks such as Tan Hill Inn — England's highest inn at 1,762 feet, and Mickle Fell, 2,591 feet — Yorkshire's highest fell, were all transferred to the newly created District. Its boundaries were clearly defined and entirely located in Durham County. The District is notably the largest unit in Durham and, in terms of population, the smallest in England; it covers an area of 208,311 acres. The river Tees ceased to serve as a natural county boundary between Yorkshire and Durham, and claimed recognition as the longest river in Durham.

The Tees, formerly known as Teisa in the twelfth century and afterwards as Teise, Teisis, Tvesis and Teyse, has retained its Celtic origin derived from T(u)is(g) meaning 'the water'. The infant Tees rises in the Cumbrian Pennine range on the southern slopes of Cross Fell, 2,930 feet, and flows 90 miles down the Pennine slopes through varied countryside to join the North Sea at Middlesbrough in Cleveland. From its source, the river drains an area of wild and desolate moorland swamped in peat bogs, until it reaches the first signs of modern civilisation at Cow Green Reservoir, then dramatically cascades 200 feet down a series of waterfalls, known as Cauldron Snout.

At this point, the Tees enters the Upper Teesdale National Nature Reserve established by the Nature Conservancy Council in September 1963, its boundaries covering an area of 8,642 acres and stretching from Cauldron Snout to High Force and south to Mickle Fell. Many footpaths cross the nature reserve and, to ensure the maintenance of fragile botanical interest, it is essential that walkers strictly adhere to the Country Code and keep to the public footpaths.

Below Cauldron Snout, the Tees joins the Maize Beck and flows between Falcon Clints and Cronkley Fell, and on to England's most impressive waterfall — High Force — where the river hurtles over the Whin Sill to fall 70 feet. It continues past Low Force to Middleton. Beyond Middleton, the river journeys through beautiful and wooded countryside, under the medieval bridge at Eggleston, and passes the charming and picturesque villages of Romaldkirk, Cotherstone and Lartington to the historic town of Barnard Castle, which is noted as the gateway to Teesdale. Downstream, the river enters 'Rokeby country' immortalised by Sir Walter Scott. The area provides many beauty spots such as Egglestone Abbey, Abbey Bridge and the 'Meeting of the Waters' and onward to Whorlton and beyond.

The surrounding countryside west of Teesdale, known as Stainmore, is drained by three main tributaries of the Tees — the Lune, Balder and Greta, as well as Deepdale Beck. This area comprising moorland and pasture includes six reservoirs which serve industrial Cleveland. Between Teesdale and Weardale is Hamsterley Forest covering 5,500 acres of forest. The Forestry Commission has created 1,100 acres of recreational area, including picnic areas, information centre, forest drive and forest walks.

Finally Teesdale is well provided with footpaths and bridleways (including 37 miles of the Pennine Way) offering unlimited variety of walks, either short or long, easy and strenuous, linking pastureland, moorland, riverside and village.

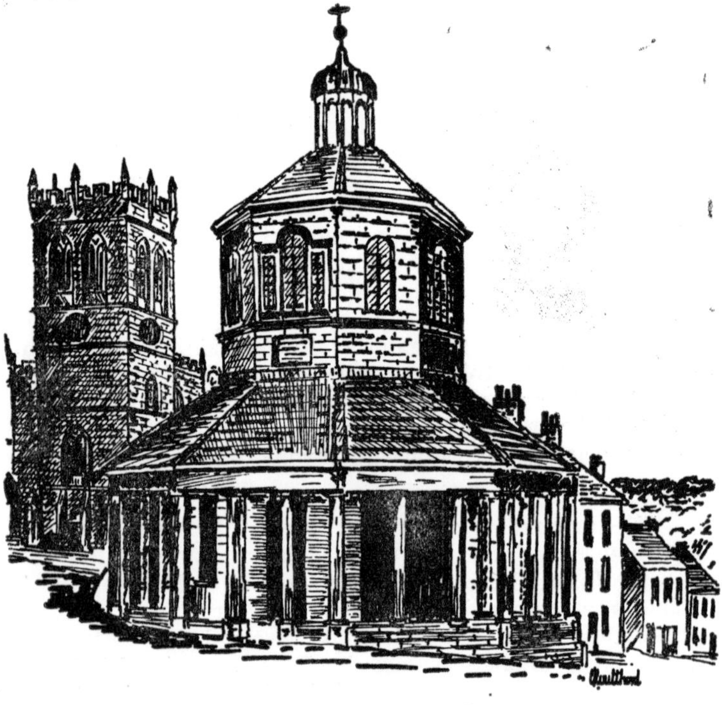

Market Cross, Barnard Castle

Part A

Walks around Barnard Castle

BARNARD CASTLE, the gateway to Teesdale, is an historic market town situated on the north bank of the river Tees, and provides an excellent starting place to explore the riverside paths, woodland and moorland areas within the very beautiful valley of Teesdale. In 1969, the town was designated a conservation area by Durham County Council, while the Council for British Archaeology listed it among 51 towns of national importance. The town is steeped in historical and literary associations providing plenty of interest for every type of visitor. It has good road communications and is well served by public transport, and there are free car parks for the motorist. It is an ideal walking centre for the rambler. The walks described in this chapter are well known and popular, providing some of the finest riverside walks in England.

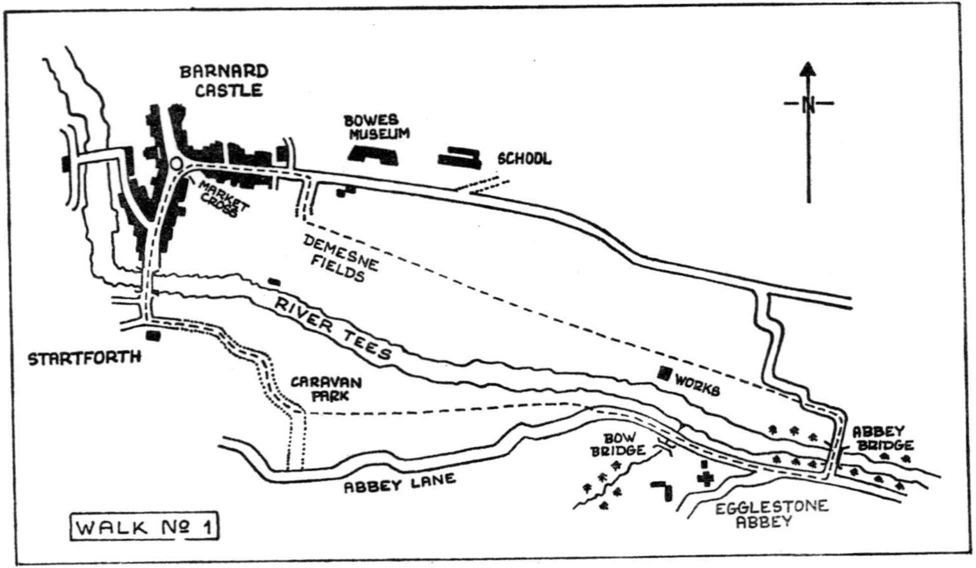

BARNARD CASTLE
BOWES MUSEUM
SCHOOL
N
MARKET CROSS
DEMESNE FIELDS
RIVER TEES
STARTFORTH
CARAVAN PARK
WORKS
ABBEY BRIDGE
BOW BRIDGE
ABBEY LANE
EGGLESTONE ABBEY
WALK No 1

1. EGGLESTONE ABBEY **Circular**

Route : Barnard Castle - The Bank - Thorngate Bridge - East Lendings Caravan Park - Egglestone Abbey - Abbey Bridge - Barnard Castle.

Distance : 3½ miles (5.6 kilometres).

Maps : One Inch — Sheet 84. 1:50 000 — Metric Sheet 92. 2½-inch — Sheet NZ01.

Car Parking : Car parks available in Barnard Castle.

Public Transport : Barnard Castle is well served with buses operated by United Automobile Services.

EGGLESTONE ABBEY is situated 1½ miles south-east of Barnard Castle and two miles north-west of Greta Bridge. The Premonstratensian abbey was dedicated to St. Mary and St. John the Baptist and founded by Ralph de Multon about 1196. The ruined abbey is preserved by the Department of Environment and admission is free. This short circular walk provides pleasant riverside scenery linked with historical associations in and around Barnard Castle. A worthwhile leaflet published by Durham County Council titled 'Walkabout — Barnard Castle' is a valuable guide and should be used in conjunction with this walk to appreciate the historic buildings of the town.

Leave Barnard Castle via Galgate, turn left into Market Place, observe the King's Head Hotel (noted for its association with Charles Dickens) and the octagonal Market Cross built in 1747. Continue down The Bank and pass Blagroves House, a 17th century house where Oliver Cromwell is said to have stayed in 1648. Pass Thorngate Mill and cross Thorngate footbridge over the Tees, where the path directly ahead climbs to The Lendings, at Startforth. Turn left along the lane to a stone stile. Cross stile, turn sharp right along the tarmac road through East Lendings caravan park and continue uphill to cross a stile on the left. Follow the well defined path, providing excellent views of Bowes Museum, to a field gate and a further two stiles to join

Abbey Lane. This delightful country lane runs parallel to the river to Bow Bridge, a 17th century pack horse bridge, now unused, where Thorsgill Beck joins the river and highlights the idyllic and graceful terrace position of Egglestone Abbey. Continue along lane to sign-post indicating 'The Abbey' which is well worth a visit. From the abbey, retrace steps to rejoin lane and road walk for 440 yards to Abbey Bridge. The former toll bridge, built in 1773, with embattled walls, is 60 feet high and has a span of 75 feet over the narrow rocky gorge of the Tees.

Cross over the bridge and walk up the road to a white kissing-gate on the left of the road. Follow field path through gate to stile and along a narrow path, where excellent views can be obtained of Egglestone Abbey; pass construction buildings of new sewerage development scheme (at time of writing), and over a stile to follow path diagonally over Demesne fields, above football playing fields, to enter Parson's Lonnen by a kissing-gate. This lane comes out opposite St. Mary's Roman Catholic church, near Bowes Museum, in Newgate. Turn left and continue along Newgate Street into the centre of Barnard Castle.

N.B.—Walks 1 and 2 can be combined to provide a 9 mile circular walk.

2. WHORLTON — Circular

Route : Whorlton - Abbey Bridge - 'Meeting of the Waters' - Whorlton.

Distance : 6 miles (9.6 kilometres).

Maps : One Inch — Sheet 84. 1:50 000 — Metric Sheet 92. 2½-inch — Sheets NZ01, NZ11.

Car Parking : There is no official car park and motorists are advised to park in the village. Please do not park on Village Green. Alternatively, parking available at Whorlton Lido on payment of fee.

Public Transport : Village is served by United Automobile Services, Route 77 (Darlington-Barnard Castle), which is an infrequent service.

WHORLTON, an attractive village, is situated south of the main Winston-Barnard Castle A67 road. The village has a fine spacious green surrounded with one-storey cottages, and the church of St. Mary re-built in 1853 has a fifty foot octagonal turret.

Leave the village and walk south towards the river Tees, pass Whorlton Court to the 'Public Footpath' sign, and turn right alongside the garden wall of Whorlton Court to enter field path route through kissing-gate. Follow path along the wooded escarpment, overlooking the Tees on the left, through fields, over two stiles and through a wooden gate. After a metal gate, there is no proper stile here, so I suggest that great care be taken to climb either the wall or fence. At this point, Sledwich Hall can be seen to the right. Keep wall on your right and descend the steps to ford Sledwich Gill. Climb out of the gill by the steps to cross a stone stile in the wall.

Follow the path above the river where the wooded banks have been extensively felled and pass through four pleasant field pastures by way of three kissing-gates and a stone stile. The path enters a large field (directly opposite the Meeting of the Waters in the distance) and the route is

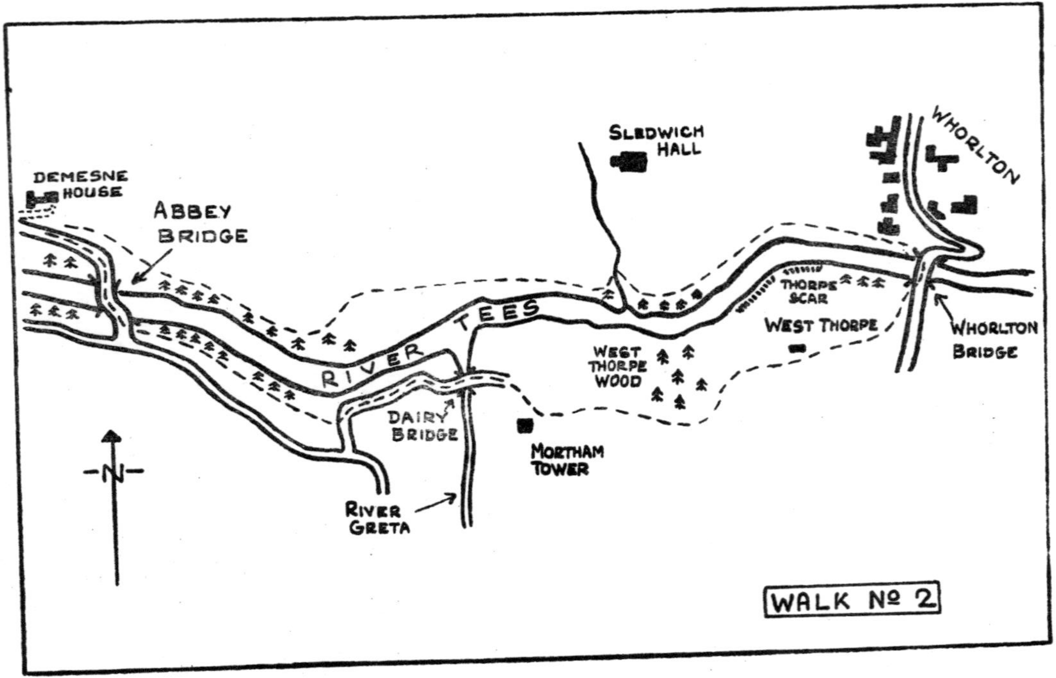
WHORLTON
SLEDWICH HALL
DEMESNE HOUSE
ABBEY BRIDGE
RIVER TEES
THORPE SCAR
WEST THORPE
WHORLTON BRIDGE
WEST THORPE WOOD
DAIRY BRIDGE
MORTHAM TOWER
RIVER GRETA
N
WALK № 2

directly ahead through a succession of stiles with the path veering to the left alongside the wood. Eventually the path enters the wood by a small wooden gate for a short distance to re-enter the field below Mains House, with the stile in the wall on the left to give access to the road. Turn left down the road and cross Abbey Bridge; immediately turn left and descend to the riverside path known as Paradise Walk. Continue along the path and cross Manyfold Beck to climb to open field above the river to enter wood by a stile. The path through the wood (overgrown during the summer months) leads to a wooden gate to reach Mortham Lane. Turn left along the lane with Rokeby Park on the right, to the Meeting of the Waters, where the river Greta joins the river Tees.

Follow cart road across Dairy Bridge over the river Greta to continue along metalled road with Mortham Tower, former 15th century peel tower, in the distance. Where the road bends, veer left to pass through a white field gate and field. Turn the corner of the field; follow the side of a small plantation and continue along path keeping by the wall on your left. The path leads to a gate by a tree; follow path with a wall on your right to a metal gate (passing building on your left known as West Thorpe). Cross field diagonally to a stile in wall opposite Whorlton Lido. Follow the road to cross Whorlton suspension bridge, which was built in 1830 and has a span of 180 feet. Immediately beyond the toll house at end of bridge, climb the steps to your left and return to the village of Whorlton.

N.B.—Walks 1 and 2 can be combined to provide a 9 mile circular walk.

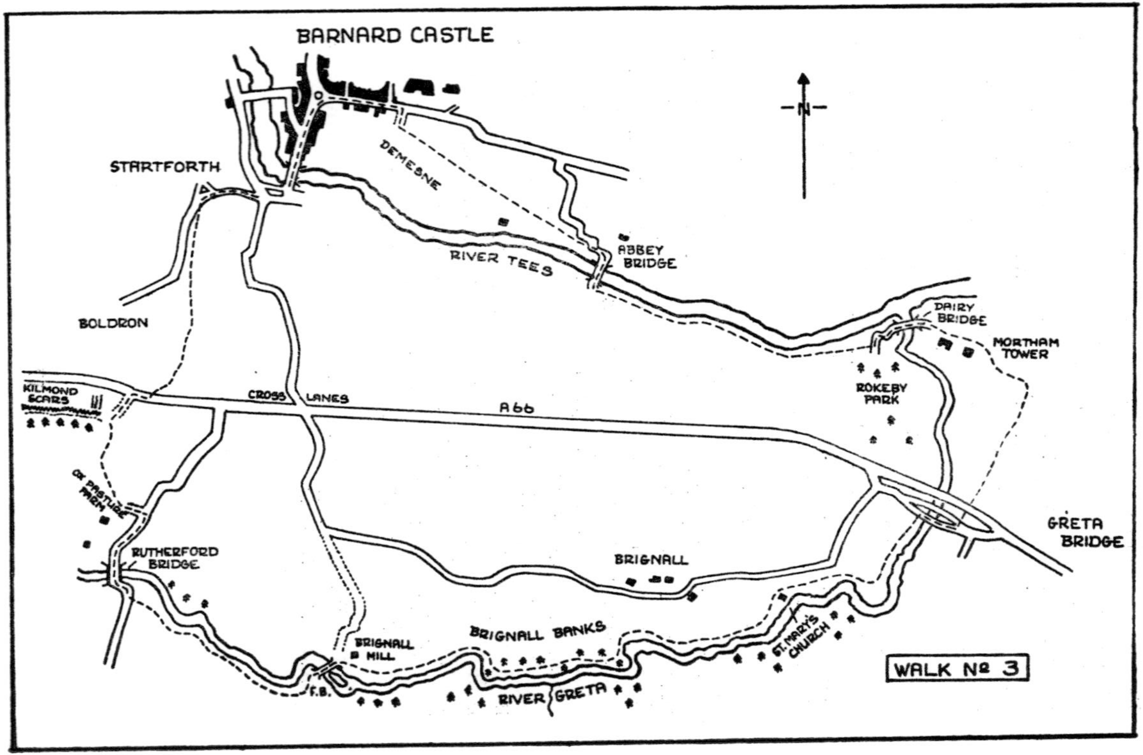
BARNARD CASTLE
N
STARTFORTH
DEMESNE
RIVER TEES
ABBEY BRIDGE
BOLDRON
DAIRY BRIDGE
NORTHAM TOWER
ROKEBY PARK
KILMOND SCARS
CROSS LANES
A66
OX PASTURE FARM
GRETA BRIDGE
RUTHERFORD BRIDGE
BRIGNALL
BRIGNALL BANKS
BRIGNALL MILL
ST. MARY'S CHURCH
F.B.
RIVER GRETA
WALK Nº 3

3. GRETADALE Circular

Route : Barnard Castle - Abbey Bridge - Mortham Tower - Greta Bridge - Brignall Mill - Rutherford Bridge - Startforth - Barnard Castle.

Distance : 11 miles (17.7 kilometres) or 7 miles (11.2 kilometres).

Maps : One Inch — Sheet 84. 1:50 000 — Metric Sheet 92. 2½-inch — Sheet NZ01.

Car Parking : Car parks available in Barnard Castle.

Public Transport : Barnard Castle is well served with buses operated by United Automobile Services. Also G.N.E. bus service from Darlington to Greta Bridge.

THE GRETA RIVER is one of the loveliest of all the tributaries of Teesdale and offers a delightful riverside walk by Brignall Banks. Sir Walter Scott described the charm and beauty of the area with his poem 'Rokeby':

O Brignall Banks are wild and fair,
And Greta Woods are green,
And you may gather garlands there
Would grace a summer queen.

This popular walk should be attempted during springtime or autumn and winter, when the woodland riverside paths can be easily negotiated in the absence of high vegetation; but, despite this recommendation, the walk is often a scramble over and under huge fallen trees, due to erosion of the banksides and heavy autumn gales. This walk is described for those walkers who are not deterred by the occasional obstruction and particularly enjoy a scramble. Its length can be reduced by using the G.N.E. bus service (Darlington to Penrith) and commencing the 7 miles walk at Greta Bridge on the A66 road.

Leave Barnard Castle via the Market Place and turn left into Newgate Street, as far as St. Mary's Roman Catholic church, just before Bowes Museum. Cross road opposite the church to enter the lane on the right, known as Parsons Lonnen, to reach Demesne Fields. Turn left, across the fields, and follow path through a number of stiles to reach the road. Follow road across Abbey Bridge and immediately turn left to descend to riverside path known as Paradise Walk, which eventually leads to Mortham Lane. Turn left along the lane, with Rokeby Park to the right, to the Meeting of the Waters, where the river Greta joins the Tees. Follow cart road across Dairy Bridge over the river Greta to walk up metalled road towards Mortham Tower, a former 15th century peel tower. Just before Mortham Tower, veer left and walk to the top corner of the field to go through gate. Continue along cart road for a hundred yards; turn right along full length of field to another gate and cross next field by a stile gradually to descend forward to the A66 road. The path is clearly sign-posted under the new A66 by-pass road bridge; cross stone stile in wall to reach the old bow bridge at Greta Bridge.

Just beyond the bridge, turn left over a low wall at the 'Public Footpath' sign and follow the path through the field banks away from the river. The path follows the woodside keeping the fence on your left and climbs to a stile. Follow path above plantation to a gate which leads into the plantation and eventually emerges into pasture land near a small stream. Continue along well defined path which descends to pass the wall of the ruined St. Mary's church (dismantled in 1833) below Brignall village. The churchyard contains memorials dated from 1676 to 1884 including tombstones to former vicars, postmasters and innkeepers of the Greta Bridge area.

Beyond the church the riverside path passes into a stretch of wood upstream. Cross another stretch of pasture to enter an extensive strip of woodland. This path is well defined and known as Brignall Banks. The path eventually climbs from the river and out of the wood to a gate and the cart road to Moor House Farm. Do not turn along this road, but descend towards the river to Brignall Mill, which has recently been restored. Cross footbridge over the Greta; turn right through the plantation to follow the riverside path. (Do not turn left beyond footbridge — this leads to Scargill). The path continues through the woodland to a second footbridge over Thwaite Beck; then forward through wooded banks and to open fields with the Greta on your right. The path emerges to ascend to a gate near 'Public Footpath' sign, and the Stang road, at Rutherford Bridge.

Turn right over the bridge and follow the road which steadily climbs passing a 'Public Footpath' sign, Bowfield and Ox Pasture Farm on the left. At the top of the hill, turn left along cart road, cross cattle grid and walk seventy yards along road, until the end of the wire fence, then veer right up a large field to a stile in wall, and onwards through further two gates to Kilmond Wood Farm. Walk through farmyard to A66 road (very busy) and cross road to a stile, which is not sign-posted, beyond the former Cross Keys Inn. The footpath is directly north, through several fields, stiles, gates, and over Thorsgill Beck. The path is easily defined and leads to the Startforth road — however, the path runs parallel to the road to Hall Farm. Walk along road through Startforth village to Thorngate Bridge over the Tees and into Barnard Castle.

N.B. : October 1978 — Ramblers' Association working party and estate workers in process of removing fallen trees and obstructions along Brignall Banks.

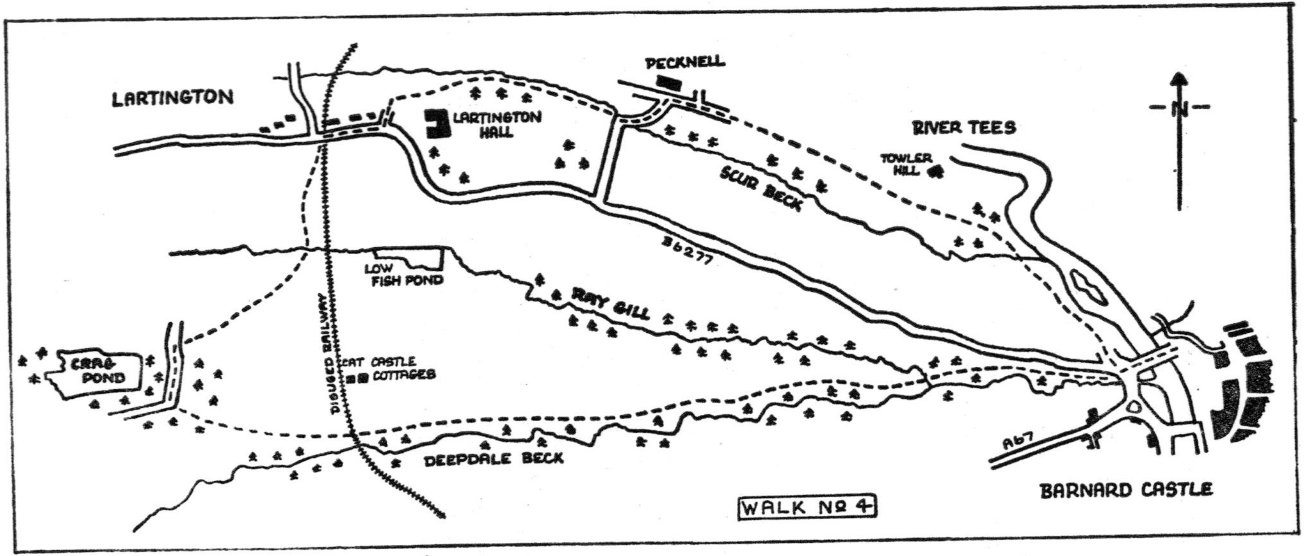
N
LARTINGTON
LARTINGTON HALL
PECKNELL
RIVER TEES
TOWLER HILL
SCUR BECK
B6277
LOW FISH POND
RAY GILL
CRAG POND
DISUSED RAILWAY
CAT CASTLE COTTAGES
DEEPDALE BECK
A67
BARNARD CASTLE
WALK Nº 4

4. DEEPDALE — Circular

Route : Barnard Castle - Deepdale - Cat Castle - Lartington - Barnard Castle.

Distance : 6 miles (9.6 kilometres).

Maps : One Inch — Sheet 84. 1:50 000 — Metric Sheet 92. 2½-inch — Sheet NZ01.

Car Parking : Car parks available in Barnard Castle.

Public Transport : Barnard Castle is well served with buses operated by United Automobile Services.

DEEPDALE, a wooded valley along Deepdale Beck, west of Barnard Castle, provides a pleasant walk through woodland scenery.

Leave Barnard Castle at bottom of Galgate, between post office and Methodist chapel. From Scar Top, take the path to the river and cross Deepdale Aqueduct footbridge over the Tees to the Barnard Castle/Lartington road — B6277. Cross road to white gate and enter Deepdale valley, a former military training area. Walk along tarmac path which follows Deepdale Beck through deciduous woodland and cross footbridge over Ray Gill, where two paths emerge — take path to left and rejoin previous route. The path continues alongside the beck to another footbridge, which spans Deepdale Beck. Do not cross bridge but follow well-defined path on the north side of beck through delightful wooded scenery abundant in bird life; one may be fortunate to catch a glimpse of the wild deer that roam this area.

Continue along a well-defined path passing the Great Stone, a huge boulder of Shap Granite situated near the beck. After three miles from the town, the path forks away from the beck and gradually climbs, often through high vegetation (which in summer months may be overgrown), to pass below the ruined buttress of the Deepdale viaduct, which once carried the South Durham and Lancashire Union Railway. The former viaduct stood 160 feet above the beck and spanned 730 feet. It was commenced on 8th October, 1857, and completed in December, 1858, at a cost of £20,687. Also, in this vicinity, are the 'cliffs of Cat Castle'; legend has it that a breed of wild cats frequented the area and that a castle actually existed. The cats have now disappeared and the castle can no longer be traced. The path levels out to pass Cat Castle quarries, now derelict, which provided local stone for the viaduct. Keep to the path high above the valley, running parallel to the wall and along the escarpment to the scar top.

Go half right through a small plantation to join cart road, with Crag Pond on the left. Turn right along the road through a gate, and right through another gate and on to The Rigg. Walk behind the farm and follow cart-road through field and, at the next field, cross diagonally to a wicket gate. Cross another field to a second wicket gate and follow small stream to the bottom of the field. Cross wooden footbridge actually wedged on the ruined stone bridge over Gill Beck and climb small slope. Continue through field in a northerly direction, keeping the fence on the left, and veer right to a stride over a wire fence at the Cat Castle Quarry access road. Enter the charming village of Lartington.

Walk the full length of the village and, at the last house called Yew Trees, turn left and follow the carriageway to a white finger post signifying the way to Barnard Castle. Continue to a second finger post through the copse, and over a stepping stile into Lartington Hall Park. Lartington Hall (former home of the Withams and built in the reign of Charles I) is to the right. Follow footpath with the Scur Beck to the left, through a gate and cross the bridge to climb the cart road with Pecknell Grange Farm to the left. Continue along cart road passing behind the cottage, to enter Pecknell Wood and cross the Scur Beck again, to follow the river Tees to the Deepdale Aqueduct and finally return to Barnard Castle.

N.B.—The disused Cat Castle Quarries were granted permission to re-open in mid-1977. Permanent stile to be erected at Cat Castle Quarry access road.

5. FLATTS WOOD Circular

Route: Barnard Castle - Scar Top - Flatts Wood - 'Rock Walk' - Barnard Castle.

Distance: 4 miles (6.4 kilometres).

Maps: One Inch — Sheet 84. 1:50 000 — Metric Sheet 92. 2½-inch — Sheet NZ01.

Car Parking: Car parks available in Barnard Castle.

Public Transport: Barnard Castle is well served with buses operated by United Automobile Services.

FLATTS WOOD, north-west of Barnard Castle, is a strip of woodland along the north bank of the river Tees which was extensively felled in the 1960s and replanted to restore its natural beauty. The wood is the property of Lord Barnard, who allows free access to walk the footpaths which were created by Dr. George Edwards over one hundred years ago. This short circular walk provides an enjoyable afternoon stroll along the wooded riverside banks of the Tees, and returns by the path above Flatts Wood.

Leave Barnard Castle via Galgate between the post office and Methodist church; and from Scar Top take the path on the left indicated by white metal sign — TO THE WOODS — to descend sharply past the Northern Gas Board holder station and follow the riverside path. Do not cross the Deepdale Aqueduct bridge, but continue along path to enter Flatts Wood, where a sign-post indicates BRIDLE PATH/FOOTPATH. Cross the newly erected footbridge over the Percy Beck and keep along the riverside path. This walk is well provided with seats which are ideal resting places to admire the riverside scenery. Further along the route another sign-post indicates FOOTPATH/BRIDLE-WAY! continue along footpath, do not ascend bridleway. The path gradually climbs to below the buttress end of the former Tees Valley viaduct which was demolished a few years ago. The viaduct was 132 feet high, built of iron and

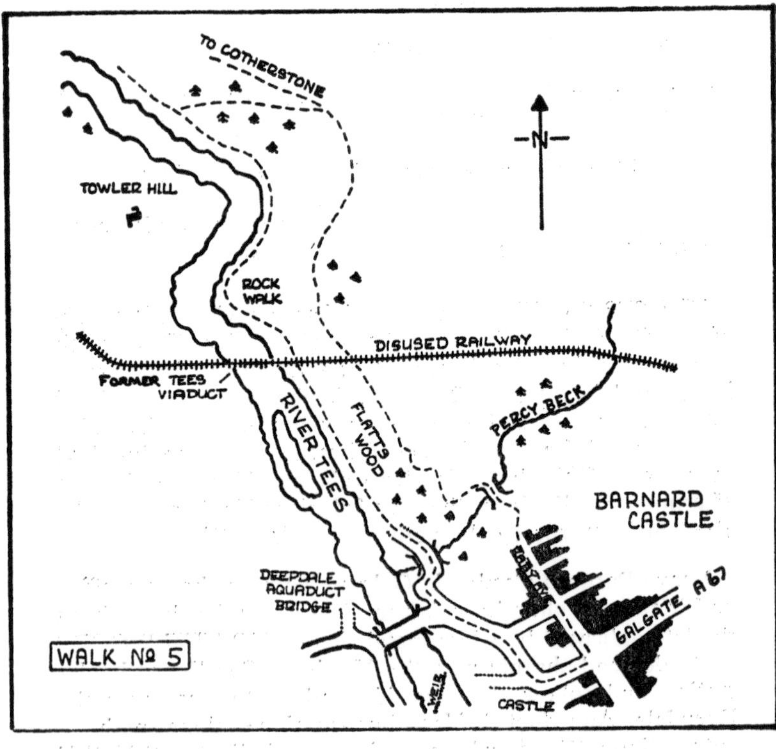
TO COTHERSTONE
N
TOWLER HILL
ROCK WALK
DISUSED RAILWAY
FORMER TEES VIADUCT
RIVER TEES
FLATTS WOOD
PERCY BECK
BARNARD CASTLE
DEEPDALE AQUADUCT BRIDGE
GALGATE A 67
WEIR
CASTLE
WALK No 5

stone at a cost of over £25,000 and had its foundation stone laid by John Wakefield on 8th October, 1857.

Pass the buttress end and continue through the wood with the path rising steeply and then gradually descending to the riverside. This part of the walk is known as the 'Rock Walk', where the Tees on the left practically encroaches the path with a rocky precipice on the right. After passing through two large boulders known as the Wishing Stones which form a stile, the path leads to a stone staircase of 29 steps. Beyond the 'Rock Walk', a small mineral spring known as 'The Spa' and noted for its medicinal waters is now difficult to locate. Even the old deer park wall is partly demolished, due to lack of preservation and it would appear that time has eluded local history of these historical features.

The path continues to a cart track on the right and leads out of the wooded valley to the open fields by a field gate above the wood. At the top, turn right and walk alongside the fence and then the wall to a wooden gate. Follow the narrow path to another gate to re-enter the open fields again.

The path continues above the wood to a field gate to cross a disused railway track (Barnard Castle-Middleton railway) near the viaduct to enter the wood. Follow the top path along the wood with the fence on the left until a hand gate is reached. Go through the gate, then turn right above the wood until a second hand gate in fence is reached. The path re-enters Flatts Wood to descend sharply to a double white sign-post which indicates TEES BANKS/ TOWN — cross wooden footbridge over the Percy Beck and climb the steps to Raby Avenue and Flatts Road to return to Barnard Castle.

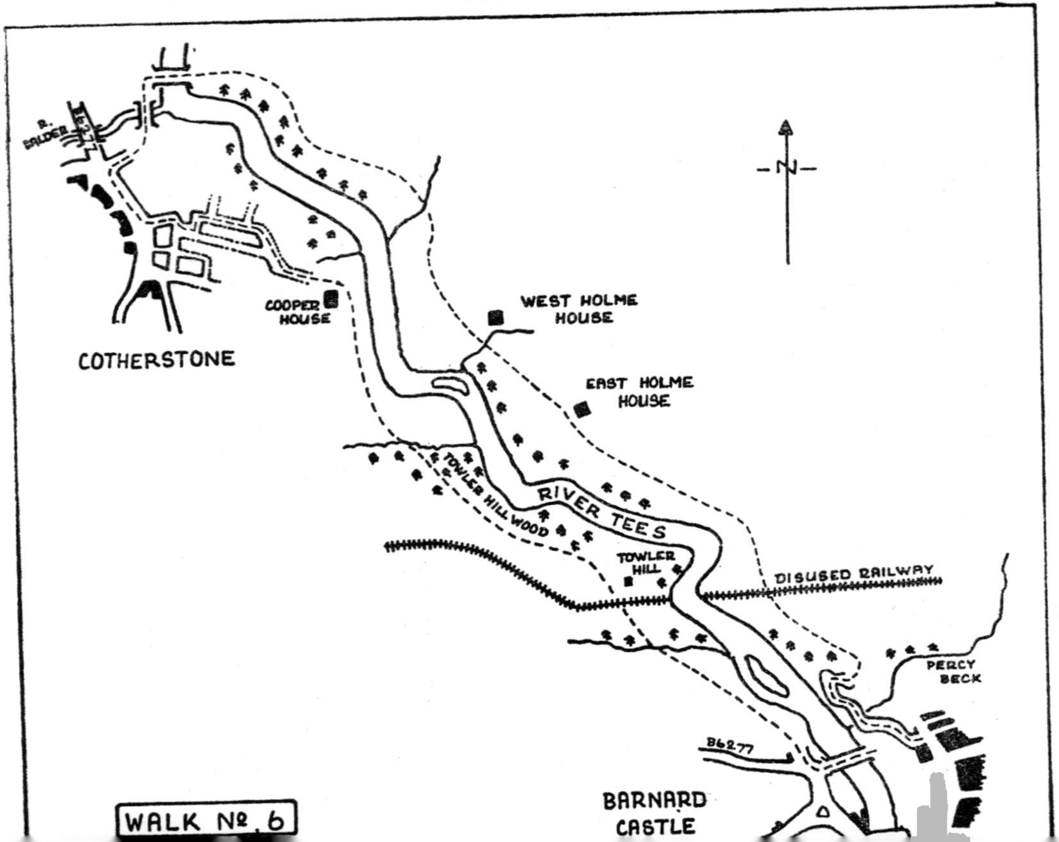

R. BALDER
B6277
COTHERSTONE
COOPER HOUSE
WEST HOLME HOUSE
EAST HOLME HOUSE
N
TOWLER HILL WOOD
RIVER TEES
TOWLER HILL
DISUSED RAILWAY
PERCY BECK
B6277
BARNARD CASTLE

WALK № 6

6. BARNARD CASTLE - COTHERSTONE Circular

Route: Barnard Castle - Flatts Wood - West Holme House - Cotherstone - Cooper House - Towler Wood - Towler Hill Farm - Barnard Castle.

Distance: 7 miles (11.2 kilometres).

Maps: One Inch — Sheet 84. 1:50 000 — Metric Sheet 92. 2½-inch — Sheets NZ01 NZ02.

Car Parking: Car parks available in Barnard Castle.

Public Transport: Barnard Castle is well served with buses operated by United Automobile Services.

THIS POPULAR WALK from Barnard Castle to Cotherstone follows the north bank of the Tees and returns along the south side of the river through pleasant pastures and riverside scenery.

This walk starts from Barnard Castle and follows the route through Flatts Wood as described in Walk 5 to the point where the track leads out of the wooded valley. At the top, turn left and keep to the fence on the left above the wood to follow the path through a couple of gates. Walk forward through a succession of four stiles adjacent metal gates to pass the white-washed farm of East Holme House on the right. The path dips to a wooden gate to West Holme House. Walk directly in front of farm, keeping farm buildings on the left to follow cart road through two fields and three gates and turn half-right across third field to a stile in fence. The narrow path descends to a stone slab footbridge across a beck and the path gradually climbs to a small gate in wall over the hill. In the distance, Cotherstone Moor, Baldersdale, and the village of Cotherstone can be seen.

Walk directly ahead to the corner of stone wall and climb to a stile in fence. Keeping the wall on the left, follow path through a small gate to a second field; cross stile and after the third field cross a stone stile in wall on the left to enter the wood above the Tees. The path gradually descends to the riverside. Follow footpath to footbridge over Tees and note two 'Public Footpath' signs, signifying paths to Barnard Castle and Low Shipley Farm respectively. Cross the footbridge and turn left along the path to cross another footbridge over the river Balder as it enters the Tees. Follow metalled path through the Hagg to enter Cotherstone opposite the Fox and Hounds.

Turn left and walk through the village to where the B6277 road bends and, directly opposite Cotherstone County Primary School, turn left into Demesne Lane, passing Bag End and Featherstone House. Follow lane (ignore two 'Public Footpath' signs) until it narrows to a stile and cross over Lane Beck. Turn left, follow outside of wood and veer right to a stile in wall and forward through a gate to Cooper House. Turn right, with the woods on your left, cross stile in wire fence and veer left to another stile adjacent a gate and farm buildings. At the next stile, observe an interesting Canadian style log cabin, and descend down the hillside to cross a beck by a stone slab bridge to a wooden stile to enter Towler Hill Wood.

The wood has recently been felled and replanted. The path is very well defined and note recent waymarking signs and posts. Follow the path uphill to cross another stile at the top, turn left and follow perimeter of field, keeping fence on your left, to a metal gate. Turn left and continue along cart road through two gates and, just before Towler Hill Farm, turn right along cart road to cross a stile in wall on the left. Follow hedgeside on your right to a stile in the corner of field and, with the wood on your left, cross a stile and the former railway embankment to descend by steps eventually to pass house on your left. Cross bridge over Scur Beck to stile adjacent gate and follow cart road to the B6277 road and return to Barnard Castle.

N.B.—Walks 6 and 8 can be combined to provide a 14 mile circular walk.

7. COTHERSTONE **Circular**

Route: Cotherstone - Balder Bridge - West End Farm - Hury Reservoir - Briscoe Lane - Cotherstone.

Distance: 6 miles (9.6 kilometres).

Maps: One Inch — Sheet 84. 1:50 000 — Metric Sheet 92. 2½-inch — Sheets NZ02, NY92, NY91.

Car Parking: Convenient parking in the village or opposite The Hagg.

Public Transport: Cotherstone is served by United Automobile Services Route 76 (Darlington-Barnard Castle-Middleton).

COTHERSTONE, formerly known as Codrestune, is situated at the junction of the rivers Balder and Tees. The village makes an excellent walking centre; it has wooded and riverside scenery with wild moorlands away to the west and rich pastoral scenes to the south and east. The walks are numerous and charming amid beautiful scenery. This walk is suitable for all; the route follows the Balder Beck and explores the smallest dale — Baldersdale.

Leave Cotherstone and walk along the main road (B6277) in a northerly direction to cross the Balder Bridge over the river Balder. Take the stone stile on your left immediately beyond the bridge; cross the field diagonally to the right and climb wooded escarpment. Follow path through six field gates, keeping the fence and strip of woodland to the left, with the Balder river below, to reach the Barnard Castle-Middleton-in-Teesdale disused railway line. Cross a pair of stepping stiles over the track and walk forward through field gate, and turn left to follow farm road to West End Farm. Pass farm buildings on your right, and immediately turn right through the farmyard and gate, then left behind the farmhouse. Continue through field to a stile in wall and make for a field gate adjacent a tree. Follow path to a stile and cross small gill, then pass a barn, keeping stone

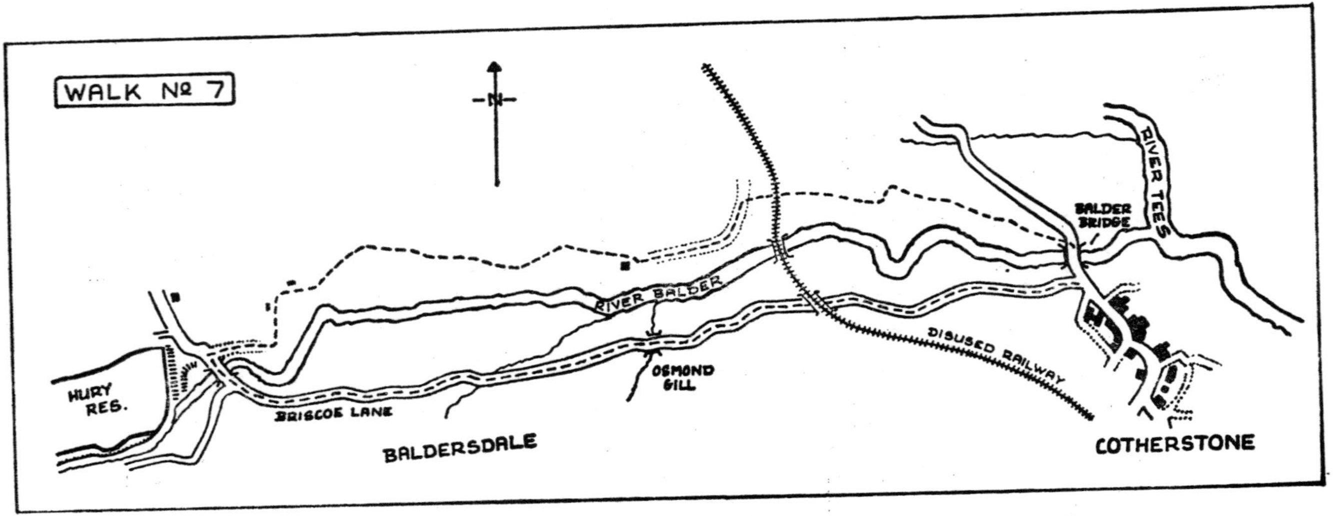
WALK № 7
N
RIVER TEES
BALDER BRIDGE
RIVER BALDER
DISUSED RAILWAY
OSMOND GILL
BRISCOE LANE
HURY RES.
BALDERSDALE
COTHERSTONE

wall on your right. The path veers left to the bottom corner of the field to cross a small footbridge over another gill. Climb the bankside, keeping the wall on the right, and continue forward passing a farm out-building on the right, then turn left in front of farmhouse. Follow farm road to reach the Hury Bridge over the Balder and to join Briscoe Lane.

At Hury Bridge, observe the spillway of the Hury reservoir, which is one of three reservoirs in Baldersdale; the other two are the Blackton and Balderhead. From the bridge, turn left to road walk along Briscoe Lane and return to Cotherstone.

N.B.—Baldersdale, which is a remote Northern Pennine valley, became well known in January 1973 after the Yorkshire Television documentary programme 'Too long a Winter' which featured the story of a remarkable woman — Miss Hannah Hauxwell of Low Birk Hatt Farm, Baldersdale. Hannah, farming alone in the Pennines, captured the imagination of the nation and since the programme she has become well known and famous. More recently, she has attended the 'Woman of the Year' luncheon at London's Savoy Hotel. *Hannah in Yorkshire* by Barry Cockcroft is published as a Dalesman paperback.

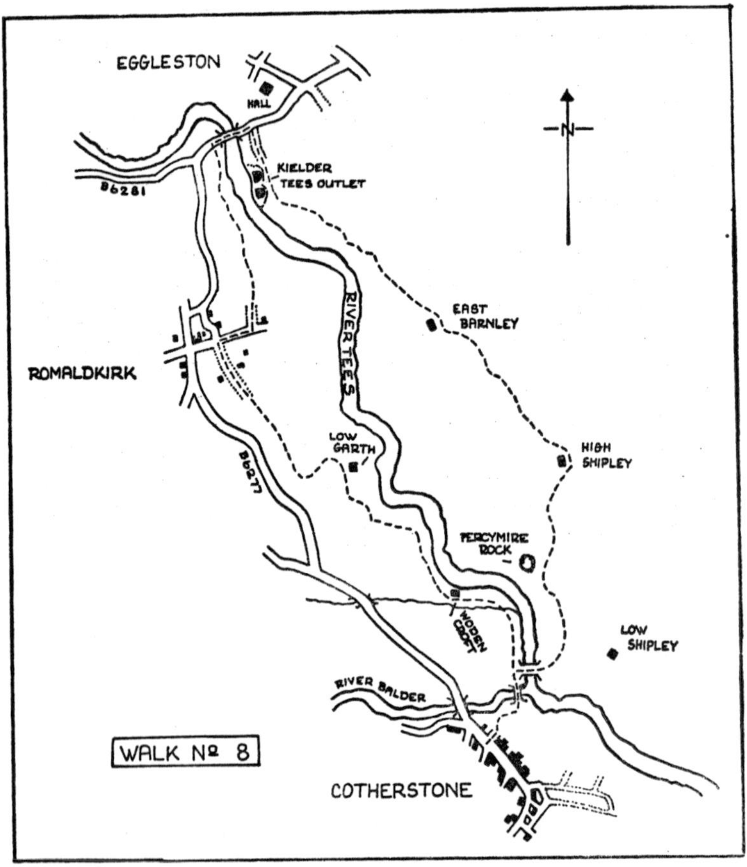
EGGLESTON
HALL
KIELDER
TEES OUTLET
B6281
EAST
BARNLEY
RIVER TEES
ROMALDKIRK
LOW
GARTH
HIGH
SHIPLEY
B6277
PERCYMIRE
ROCK
WODEN
CROFT
LOW
SHIPLEY
RIVER BALDER
WALK No 8
COTHERSTONE

8. ROMALDKIRK **Circular**

Route: Romaldkirk - Eggleston Bridge - High Shipley - Cotherstone - Woden Croft - Romaldkirk.

Distance: 7 miles (11.2 kilometres).

Maps: One Inch — Sheet 84. 1:50 000 — Metric Sheet 92. 2½-inch — Sheets NY92, NZ02.

Car Parking: Convenient parking in village: please do not park on village green.

Public Transport: Romaldkirk is served by United Automobile Services Route 76 (Darlington-Barnard Castle-Middleton).

ROMALDKIRK is one of the prettiest villages in Teesdale, with a spacious green, an old water pump, stocks and the church of St. Romald, which is regarded as the 'Cathedral of the Dale'.

Walk to the bottom of the village passing the church and, immediately beyond Beck Wharfe, turn left at 'Public Footpath' sign, along narrow green lane to cross stone footbridge over Beer Beck. Follow lane to stone stile on the left and take path to stone stile on the right (ignore gap in wall and gate near cemetery) to climb gradually over Hewcroft Hill; Eggleston Hall can be seen in the distance. Cross field diagonally to a recently built wall and follow path to stile above the lovely wooded banks of the Tees. Continue towards gate by stone building with 'Public Footpath' sign to B6281 road by Eggleston Bridge.

Cross the medieval bridge where a chapel once stood at the southern approach. Immediately beyond the bridge observe a 'Public Footpath' sign and, next to it, a Northumbrian Water Authority notice — 'Tyne Tees Tunnelling Tees Valley Works', indicating the Kielder water scheme (Tees outlet). Follow metalled road to construction site.

The Kielder scheme is to link the reservoir with the region's main rivers — the Derwent, the Wear and the Tees. This involves digging huge underground tunnels joining the rivers, with the Wear outlet near Frosterley and the Tees outlet near Eggleston. Nearly 32 kilometres (20 miles) of the aqueduct will be in tunnels of 2.9 metres (9.5 feet) diameter.

Follow diversion route (in operation at the time of writing), which is well defined by tapes and footpath signs, to cross over two footbridges directly above the two aqueduct tunnels. Immediately after second bridge, climb sharp incline on the left, through the wood above to a wooden gate in the corner of the wall. (Do not continue along riverside path which is a private path). Proceed diagonally across field to a stile and onward to gate in corner of field to East Barnley Farm. Walk behind the farmhouse along cart road to gate in wall. The path continues across next field and gradually climbs to 900 feet, passing Raygill Beck, to a stone stile in wall. Proceed across further field to join small plantation and cart road through High Shipley Farm — a former 17th century farmhouse and hunting lodge of James II. (Note the inscription E.G.S. for Eunice and George Simpson — 1670 — with stag and hounds carved over the mullion window).

Leave farm and turn right through gate adjacent plantation to descend diagonally across field to stile in corner of wall. Cross stream (often muddy) and proceed downwards to gate and onwards to stile in wall to reach the elevated position of Percymire Rock (approx. 900 feet above sea level), which offers excellent views overlooking Cotherstone and Baldersdale — Goldsborough (1,247 feet) and Shacklesborough (1,489 feet). From the 'Rock' continue over small bridge to stile in corner of wall and follow path with beck on right to another stile. Descend through gorse bushes to caravan site and take broad track through the site to the river and cross bridge over the Tees. Do not turn left or cross bridge over the river Balder unless you wish to explore Cotherstone.

Turn right over the bridge and follow riverside path to cross stile in wall and enter field to a further stile to negotiate stepping stones over Wildon Beck. The path gradually climbs and veers away from the river to a gate and onwards to Woden Croft (former Dotheboys School). Pass in front of farm; go through farmyard to a gate, and stile, to continue along path keeping wood on your right to another gate. Take the next gate on your right to enter the wood and see the Fairy Cupboards which are rock indentations in the riverside.

Retrace your steps to gate and walk diagonally across field and through another gate to pass a building regarded as a resting place for the monks travelling between Egglestone Abbey and Romaldkirk. Follow path by fence on the right above the wood to a gate, and proceed towards Low Garth Farm crossing a stile, two streams and going through two field gates. From farm, follow cart road to a wicket gate in the hedge on the right and cross field diagonally to another wicket gate in corner of field: continue in the same direction to two gates side by side and take the gate on the right to enter Sennings Lane. Follow lane and return to Romaldkirk.

N.B.—Walks 6 and 8 can be combined to provide a 14 mile circular walk.

Part B

Walks around Middleton-in-Teesdale

MIDDLETON-IN-TEESDALE, the capital of Upper Teesdale and former administrative headquarters of the London Lead Company, is situated on the north bank of the Tees. The town is an ideal centre for walkers with the commencement of several fine walks on both sides of the river, including the Pennine Way along the south bank. It is the starting point for High Force and Cauldron Snout waterfalls, and the wild and romantic scenery of the upper reaches of the Tees.

9. KIRK CARRION **Circular**

Route: Middleton - Kirk Carrion - Bowbank - Laithkirk - Middleton.

Distance: 5 miles (8.0 kilometres).

Maps: One Inch — Sheet 84. 1:50 000 — Metric Sheet 92. 2½-inch — Sheet NY92.

Car Parking: Car park available in Middleton-in-Teesdale.

Public Transport: Middleton is served by United Automobile Services Route 76 (Darlington - Barnard Castle - Middleton).

KIRK CARRION is a clump of trees and prominent landmark situated on Bowbank Fell, south of Middleton-in-Teesdale and overlooking the valley. The trees mark the site of a great tumulus which, when opened in 1804, was found to contain a small cinerary urn and fragments of bone believed to be that of a Brigantes prince called Caryn. The burial ground is reputed to be haunted.

Leave Middleton by the B6277 road and walk south over Middleton Bridge across the Tees. Pass cattle mart on the right to the Holwick road junction. Turn right and, immediately opposite the Gate House, turn left through a gate adjacent bridleway sign and climb the steep hill. Follow the well-defined green track, passing through two gates and onwards in the general direction towards the clump of trees ahead. However, the right of way is through a metal gate in a stone wall to the left. (While there is evidence of a well worn track following the boundary wall ascending to Kirk Carrion, this is not a right of way, but obviously popular with walkers and well worth the visit). Retrace steps to original route and, in the distance, observe the Grassholme reservoir in Lunedale. The path descends to a gate in wall and joins the B6276 Lunedale road.

Turn left along the narrow road (great care should be taken when road walking) which is a popular motorists' route for those using the recreational facilities provided by the Northumbrian Water Authority at the Lunedale reservoirs. Follow the road, passing the small hamlet of Bowbank, and at the road junction turn right; on the left, at the

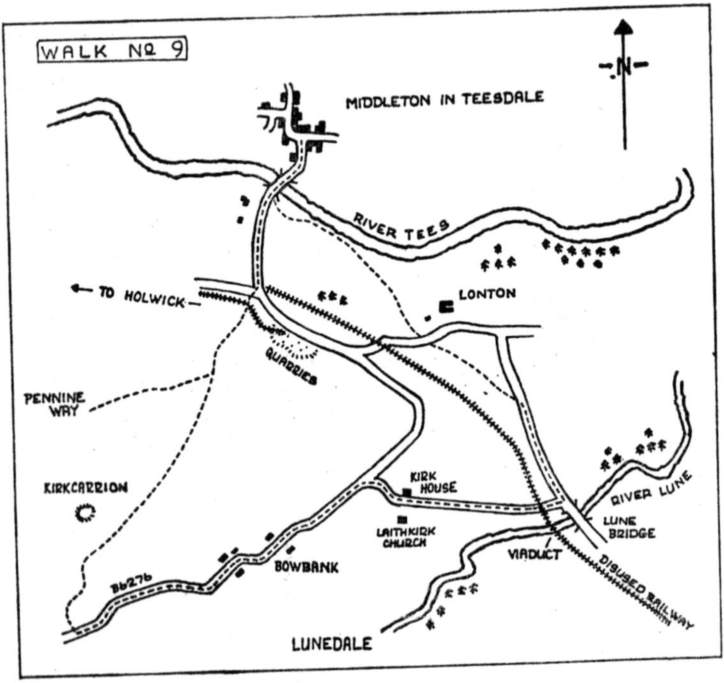
WALK No 9
N
MIDDLETON IN TEESDALE
RIVER TEES
TO HOLWICK
LONTON
QUARRIES
PENNINE WAY
KIRKCARRION
KIRK HOUSE
RIVER LUNE
LUNE BRIDGE
LAITHKIRK CHURCH
VIADUCT
BOWBANK
B6276
DISUSED RAILWAY
LUNEDALE

top of Laithkirk Bank, is Kirk House, a former wayside inn. Note the inscription on its wall:

Good Ale
Pipes and
Tobacco:
If by you go,
And dry you be,
The fault's in you
And not in me.

On the opposite side of the road is the Church of the Holy Barn — Laithkirk church. Formerly Lord Fitzhurgh's tithe-barn, it is one of the most primitive of churches and has been used as a consecrated building since the 15th century.

Follow the road down Laithkirk Bank with the river Lune on the right to pass under the Lune viaduct. At the road junction, turn left and follow the B6277 road for a few hundred yards to a stile on the left. Cross field (note disused Middleton-Barnard Castle railway line to your left) to rejoin the road near Lonton South Farm. Take stile on the right of the road and follow defined path through a succession of fields and stiles, passing Step Ends, and along cart road to walk alongside the Tees to the footsteps at Middleton Bridge. Turn right and follow road into Middleton.

Route: Middleton - Scoberry Bridge - Newbiggin - Middleton.

Distance: 6 miles (9.7 kilometres).

Maps: One Inch — Sheet 84. 1:50 000 — Metric Sheets 92 or 91. 2½-inch — Sheet NY92.

Car Parking: Car park available in Middleton-in-Teesdale.

Public Transport: Middleton is served by United Automobile Services Route 76 (Darlington-Barnard Castle-Middleton).

LEAVE MIDDLETON by the B6277 road and walk south over Middleton Bridge across the Tees. Immediately beyond the cattle mart at the 'Public Footpath' sign, leave the road to cross stile and follow the cart road on the south side of the Tees. This footpath is part of the Pennine Way which passes through some of the finest river scenery in England. The way is well defined and easy to follow due to the popularity of this long-distance walk.

The cart road running parallel to the river Tees passes through numerous stiled field pastures and leads into a narrow walled lane — part of the Old Holwick Road which was an ancient way from Laithkirk to Holwick. The path leaves the river to cross Unthank Beck, passing the edge of Park End Wood, a remnant of the Teesdale natural forest, and climbs Unthank Bank near the site of the haunted hamlet of Unthank. Beyond the hill, care must be taken to descend the steep wooded bank to cross the footbridge over Holwick Beck, where the former stepping stones are visible. Cross over two ladder stiles; the path keeps close to the river bank to Scoberry Bridge, the link between Holwick and Newbiggin. Near the bridge is the narrow rocky channel known as 'The Leap'.

Cross Scoberry Bridge over the Tees, and go through two fields; cross footbridge over the Bowlees Beck and walk forward along a narrow walled path to cross field to stile,

'Public Footpath' sign and Middleton Road (B6277). Cross road and follow lane into Newbiggin. Walk to the east end of the village, passing behind the Methodist chapel which was founded 200 years ago when John Wesley preached here. Follow Miry Lane, which climbs up the hillside to pass Corner Cottage on the left and zig zags to meet the Middleside road. Turn right and walk along this quiet and pleasant road and observe the wonderful views across the valley, including Kirk Carrion, Crossthwaite Moor, Holwick Scar and Cronkley Fell. Follow the road for two miles, gradually descending to pass Bell's Farm, Middleside and Lanehead. Middleton House, former headquarters of the London Lead Company, is at the top of the Hude. Descend steeply to Hudeshope Bridge and enter the Market Place at Middleton-in-Teesdale.

N.B.—Walks 10, 11 (part route) and 12 (part route) can be combined to provide an 11 mile circular walk. See combined map on page 44.

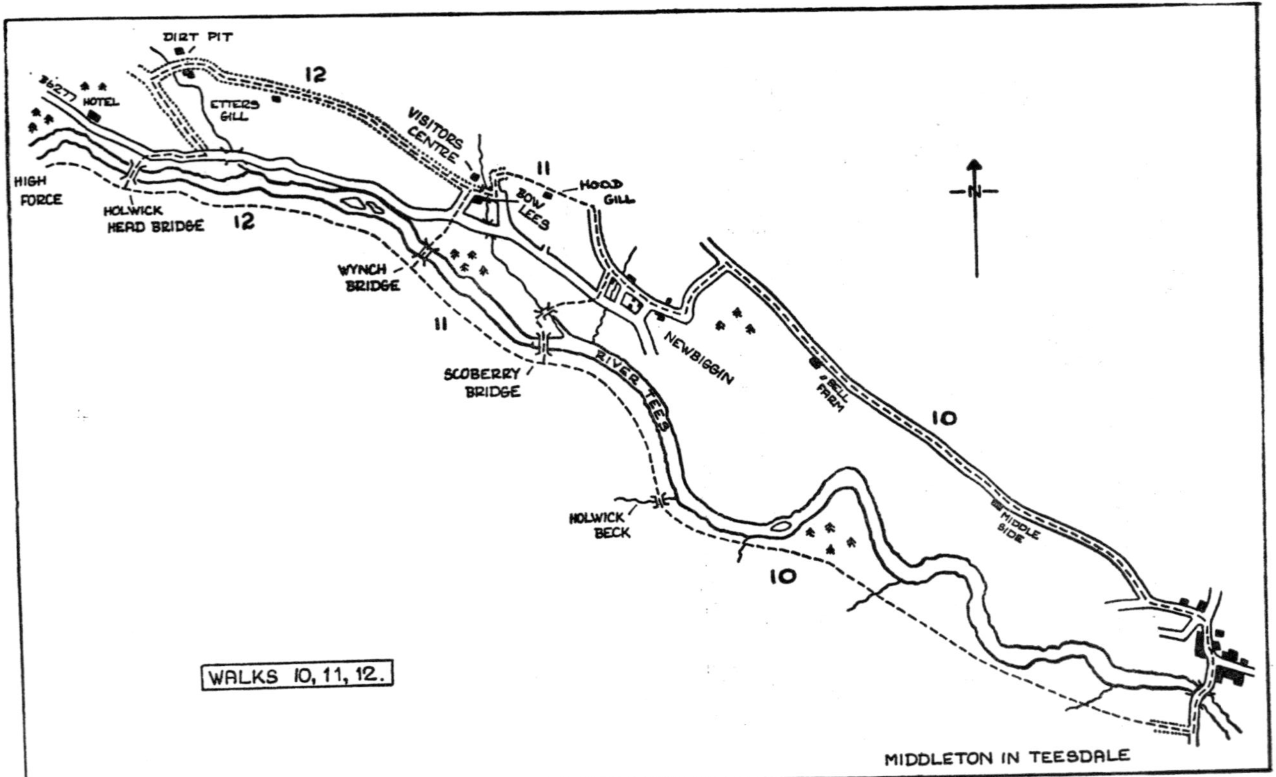
DIRT PIT
12
B6277
HOTEL
ETTERS GILL
VISITORS CENTRE
11
HOOD GILL
BOW LEES
HIGH FORCE
HOLWICK HEAD BRIDGE
12
WYNCH BRIDGE
11
NEWBIGGIN
BELL FARM
SCOBERRY BRIDGE
RIVER TEES
10
N
HOLWICK BECK
MIDDLE SIDE
10
WALKS 10, 11, 12.
MIDDLETON IN TEESDALE

11. BOWLEES — 1 Circular

Route : Bowlees - Hood Gill - Newbiggin - Scoberry Bridge - Wynch Bridge - Low Force - Bowlees.

Distance : 2 miles (3.2 kilometres).

Maps : One Inch — Sheet 84. 1:50 000 — Metric Sheets 92, 91. 2½-inch — Sheet NY92.

Car Parking : Bowlees Picnic Area G.R. 908282.

Public Transport :

1. *United Automobile Services Route 76 (Barnard Castle-High Force — Summer only). Please check bus timetable.*
2. *Teesdale Coach Services Route 115 (Barnard Castle-Langdon Beck.) Please check bus timetable.*

BOWLEES, meaning 'the clearing at the bend of the hills', is a small hamlet of six terrace houses, a bungalow, a farm and a former Methodist chapel. This hamlet is situated north of the B6277 road, midway between Middleton-in-Teesdale and High Force. North-East of Bowlees, G.R. 908282, a disused quarry has been developed by Durham County Council and laid out as a picnic area, through which Bowlees Beck flows from Swinhope Head. It is an ideal beauty spot for the family, with parking places, toilets, picnic tables, play area for children, and nature trail. A warden's hut is used as an information centre, which is manned by Durham Countryside Rangers on summer week-ends. The site is ideally located and promises to be one of Durham's most attractive picnic areas, with Gibson's Cave, ¼ mile north along Bowlees Beck; Low Force and Wynch Bridge, ½ mile south-west; and, eighty yards beyond the ford, the Durham County Conservation Trust Visitors' Centre, located in the converted Primitive Methodist chapel. The Centre was officially opened in July 1976; it is open from Easter to October (admission fee) and provides information, exhibits and displays relating to past and present Teesdale. It is well worth a visit.

Follow the new footpath for ¼ mile upstream alongside Bowlees Beck to Gibson's Cave (this is not a right of way but the Raby Estates have kindly given permission for public access). Here, due to the action of a 20 foot waterfall (called Summery Hill Force), the hard limestone shelf has been worn away to create a 'cave'. Return to picnic area.

Leave picnic area through gate by cattle grid marked 'no exit', follow cart road and turn right where this road bends sharp left. Walk across field to gate, and through a second field to pass behind a row of houses known as Hood Gill to two stiles adjacent gates. Continue along green track; pass stone building on the left and, keeping the wire fence on your right, reach a stile adjacent gate. Follow field path to stile adjacent another gate near a 'Public Footpath' sign. Turn right and descend downhill into Newbiggin.

Follow lane between Fellowship Farm and Chapel View to B6277 road junction. Turn right and cross the main road to a 'Public Footpath' sign and stile on your left. Proceed diagonally across the field to a stile in the corner of field; walk down narrow enclosed path, ignore stile on the left, and cross footbridge over Bowlees Beck. Cross field and, keeping the building on your right, proceed forward to Scoberry Bridge. Cross bridge over the Tees and turn right to follow the well defined path along the river, which is part of the Pennine Way. Ignore stile on your left which is the path to Holwick.

Continue along riverside path; cross a newly erected footbridge over a small beck and follow path to Wynch Bridge, a suspension bridge over the Tees. Turn right and cross over the bridge; observe the Low Force waterfalls. Proceed forward through wood to a stile and cross two fields to a 'Public Footpath' sign and the B6277 road. Follow lane into Bowlees, passing the Visitors' Centre, and return to the picnic area.

N.B.—Walks 10, 11 and 12, see combined map on page 44.

12. BOWLEES — 2 Circular

Route: Bowlees - Ash Hill - Dirt Pit - Holwick Head Bridge - High Force - Wynch Bridge - Bowlees.

Distance: 5 miles (8.0 kilometres) — including extension to High Force.

Maps: One Inch — Sheet 84. 1:50 000 — Metric Sheets 92, 91. 2½-inch — Sheet NY92.

Car Parking: Bowlees Picnic Area G.R. 908282.

Public Transport:

1. United Automobile Services Route 76 (Barnard Castle-High Force — Summer only, infrequent service).

2. Teesdale Coach Services Route 115 (Middleton-Langdon Beck — infrequent service.) Please check bus timetable.

THIS SECOND WALK from Bowlees also starts from the picnic area, and the visitor should cross the ford over Bowlees Beck and walk along the new footpath passing the Visitors' Centre on the right. Near the Centre, a 'Public Footpath' sign on the left indicates the Old Road (Forest to Middleton) which should be followed. Gradually ascend through numerous fields and gates to pass Ash Hill on the left. From this point extensive views up and down the valley can be obtained. The road gradually descends to Dirt Pit, formerly known as 'Durpit' or 'Deerpath', meaning a deer path when deer roamed the Teesdale Forest.

Walk between the cottages and farmhouses to cross the bridge over Ettersgill Beck; turn left along the road until it reaches the B6277 (Middleton-Alston road). Turn right for a few yards to cross the road and descend a narrow lane on your left to the wooden Holwick Head Bridge over the Tees.

From this point, I recommend the extension walk to High Force. Turn right and climb the hill below Holwick Head House to the fell gate and enter the Upper Teesdale National Nature Reserve — please keep to the path and observe the Country Code. The path winds through juniper bushes (which probably form the most extensive juniper forest to survive in England). Pass through two kissing-gates and over stepping boards (installed by the Nature Conservancy Council with financial assistance from the Countryside Commission) to negotiate the muddy stretches in order to reach the gorge and High Force waterfall.

To return, retrace your steps to pass Holwick Head Bridge on your left, and follow the defined path along the Pennine Way for one mile. Pass Low Force, which is a popular picnic spot, to reach Wynch Bridge. Cross the suspension bridge, which provides an excellent viewpoint of Low Force or Salmon Leap directly above, while downstream Staple Crag is a detached massive rock of whinstone.

According to C. P. Nicholson's *Teesdale* Handy Guide Series: 'It is said to have been the earliest suspension bridge in England and possibly in Europe. It was 60 feet long and hung 21 feet above the river — the present suspension bridge was erected in 1830.' In November 1771 it was severely damaged by the great flood and, on 20th August 1802, one of the main chains collapsed as a party of haymakers was returning from Holwick. Two men were hurled into the river below and an 18 year old youth was drowned.

Proceed forward through wood to a stile and cross two fields to a 'Public Footpath' sign and the B6277 road. Follow lane into Bowlees, passing the Visitors' Centre, and return to the picnic area.

N.B.—Walks 10, 11 and 12, see combined map on page 44.

13. COW GREEN RESERVOIR Circular

Route : Weelhead Sike Car Park - Cauldron Snout - Falcon Clints - Widdybank Farm - Peghorn Lane - Weelhead Sike Car Park.

Distance : Approx. 8 miles (including extension to Langdon Beck Hotel) (12.8 kilometres).

Maps : One Inch — Sheet 84. 1:50 000 — Metric Sheets 92, 91. 2½-inch — Sheets NY83, NY82.

Car Parking : Weelhead Sike Car Park, Peghorn Lane — G.R. 811310.

COW GREEN RESERVOIR, costing £2½m., was completed in 1970 and officially opened on 22nd July, 1971. It is the biggest reservoir in Teesdale, covering a surface of 770 acres and holding 9,000 million gallons of water by a dam 82 feet high and 623 yards long. The reservoir was built despite strong opposition from conservationists, including the Ramblers' Association.

From Weelhead Sike car park, walk along Peghorn Lane in an easterly direction for a few yards. Turn right by the stone cairn to follow the old miners' way and then go through the kissing-gate to enter the Upper Teesdale National Nature Reserve. Follow the footpath to Cauldron Snout — one of England's finest waterfalls (please do not stray from this route). To the west, the reservoir can be observed and it is interesting to note how it has naturally blended with the moorland scenery.

On reaching the head of the waterfall, a new bridge over the Tees — situated yards below the dam head — points the way to Birkdale Farm, High Cup Nick and the Eden Valley. However, the route is down the eastern side of the waterfall and real care must be taken when descending the rocky staircase which is often slippery in wet weather. At the foot, one can admire this 200 foot waterfall which is a most impressive sight. The walk has now encountered the

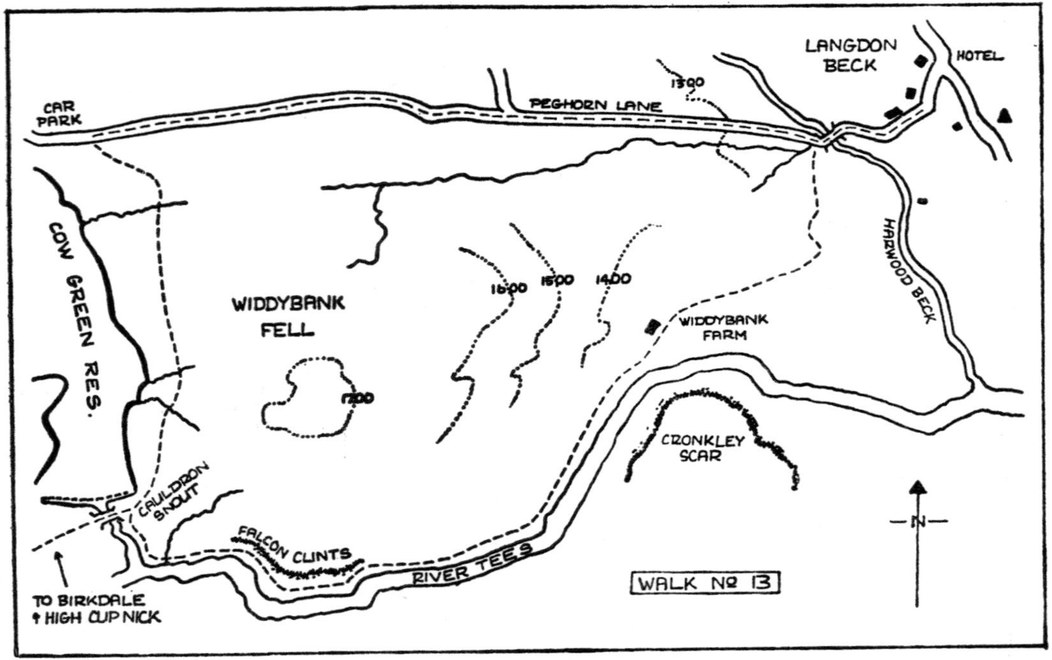
LANGDON BECK
HOTEL
CAR PARK
PEGHORN LANE
1300
HARWOOD BECK
1400
1500
1600
WIDDYBANK FARM
WIDDYBANK FELL
1700
COW GREEN RES.
CAULDRON SNOUT
FALCON CLINTS
RIVER TEES
CRONKLEY SCAR
N
WALK № 13
TO BIRKDALE & HIGH CUP NICK

Pennine Way along the north bank of the Tees. Some distance below the waterfall, the Tees is joined by the Maize Beck — a former meeting place of Yorkshire, Durham and Westmorland.

Follow the Tees downstream by a path which winds its way below the high basaltic cliffs of Falcon Clints, at the edge of Widdybank Fell. This section of the walk is often boggy in wet weather and, to overcome this difficulty, walkers are advised to wear strong footwear — even though the Nature Conservancy Council have installed stepping boards (with financial assistance from the Countryside Commission) along this stretch. Further on, the path becomes narrow and rougher and the walker must negotiate large boulders and scree to reach the pleasant pastures of Holmwath, overlooked by the dark cliffs of Cronkley Scar. The path leads to a high wall stile and over a sike by stepping boards to Widdybank Farm — notably the first inhabitation near the Tees.

Below Cronkley Scar, on the south bank of the river, is an old ruined pencil mill. The now exhausted outcrop of soft slate was once worked for the making of slate pencils, known in the district as "Widdies."

Follow path through farmyard — please observe request to keep to the path — and continue along rough cart-road over the fell. Ahead, we see the whitewashed farmsteads of the Langdon Beck area, which are so typical of the Teesdale valley north of the river and form part of the Raby Estates. The farms are white as stipulated in their leases, and the reasons for this are associated with two local country tales. One tale states that a former Lord Barnard was refused a glass of milk at a lonely farm and afterwards decided that, in order to recognise his tenancies, all properties should be whitewashed annually. The second tale states similarly that a former Lord Barnard sought refuge overnight at a lonely farmhouse and, in return for the kind hospitality, agreed to pay for repairs to the property. However, on receipt of the heavy bill, Lord Barnard was shocked to learn that the farm was not part of his estates and immediately decreed that all his farms should be whitewashed annually.

To continue, follow cart-road for a mile to join Peghorn Lane. Time permitting, walkers may obtain refreshments at Langdon Beck Hotel and should turn right along Peghorn Lane, crossing the bridge over the Harwood Beck to the hotel. Alternatively, to complete the walk, turn left along Peghorn Lane — a former miners' track — and gradually climb the metalled road for 2½ miles to return to the car park.

Part C

Hostel to Hostel

YOUTH HOSTELLING provides an interesting way for hostellers to explore Upper Teesdale. Often guide books tend to omit walks especially for youth hostellers and, for this reason, Hostel to Hostel walks have been included, chiefly for the experienced hosteller/walker and Pennine Way walker. Walks between Barnard Castle, Langdon Beck and Dufton Youth Hostels link Teesdale with the Upper Eden Valley.

Further details regarding the Youth Hostels' Association should be obtained from Trevelyan House, 8 St. Stephens Hill, St. Albans, Herts, AL1 2DY. The regional handbook — *Border and Dales* — provides very useful information.

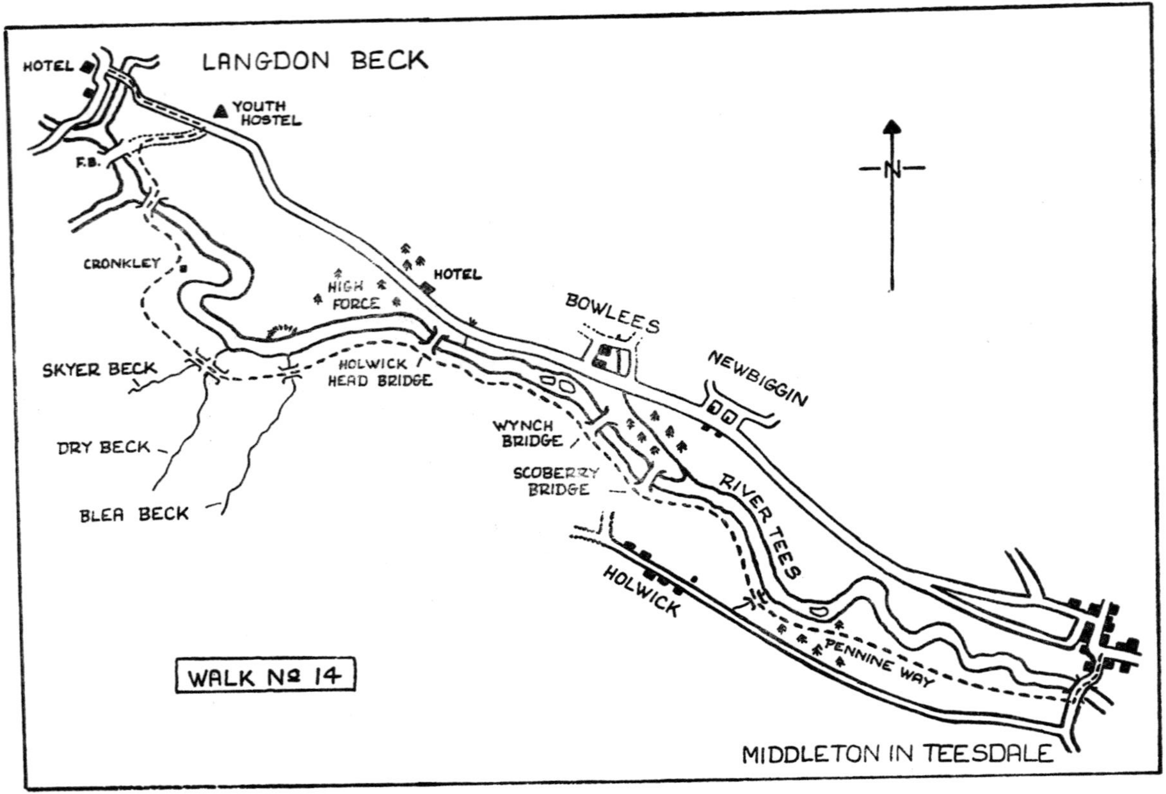
LANGDON BECK
HOTEL
YOUTH HOSTEL
F.B.
N
CRONKLEY
HIGH FORCE
HOTEL
BOWLEES
NEWBIGGIN
SKYER BECK
HOLWICK HEAD BRIDGE
DRY BECK
WYNCH BRIDGE
SCOBERRY BRIDGE
BLEA BECK
RIVER TEES
HOLWICK
PENNINE WAY
WALK No 14
MIDDLETON IN TEESDALE

14. MIDDLETON - LANGDON BECK Non-Circular

Route: Middleton - High Force - Cronkley Bridge - Langdon Beck Youth Hostel.

Distance: 7 miles (11.2 kilometres) or 17 miles (27.2 kilometres).

Maps: One Inch — Sheet 84. 1:50 000 — Metric Sheets 92, 91. 2½-inch — Sheets NZ01, NZ02, NY92, NY82, NY83.

Public Transport: Middleton is served by United Automobile Services Route 76 (Darlington-Barnard Castle-Middleton).

AFTER AN ENJOYABLE stay at Barnard Castle Youth Hostel, my companion and I, on this occasion, decided to travel by bus from Barnard Castle to Middleton-in-Teesdale, rather than attempt the full distance of 17 miles between Barnard Castle and Langdon Beck Youth Hostels. The youth hosteller is well advised and recommended to do likewise, and undertake the shorter walk of 7 miles between Middleton to Langdon Beck Youth Hostel.

However, those hostellers wishing to attempt the full length of the walk should carefully plan the route; allow plenty of time to undertake the walk, consider weather conditions, and have an adequate knowledge of map-reading.

Walks 5, 6 and 8 (part of route) outlined in the book should provide sufficient guidance for the walker to reach East Barnley Farm. From this farm, follow the defined path to West Barnley to reach the B6281 (Eggleston-Middleton road). Turn left by 'Public Footpath' sign and walk along B6282 road for approximately 1¼ miles to turn left into lane, opposite Egglesburn House, towards Toby Hill Farm and above Ornelly Farm. Follow the riverside path through numerous fields to Middleton Bridge and into Middleton-in-Teesdale. This little town is worth visiting for refreshments and is regarded as the capital of Upper Teesdale. (Note the Bainbridge Memorial Fountain, a link with the former lead mining industry).

I make no apology or excuse for repeating part of this second stage of the walk, as outlined in Walks 10, 11 and 12 (part routes), as I personally regard this walk as the finest riverside scenery in England.

Leave Middleton by the B6277 road and walk south over Middleton Bridge across the Tees. Immediately beyond the cattle mart at the 'Public Footpath' sign, leave the road to cross a stile and follow the cart-road on the south side of the Tees. This footpath is the Pennine Way. Follow the Way in a westerly direction alongside the Tees through numerous stiled field pastures to reach the first of four main footbridges over the river — Scoberry Bridge. Do not cross this bridge, but continue along the well-defined path and, just before Wynch Bridge, observe Holwick Lodge, below Holwick Scars, a shooting lodge owned by the Earl of Strathmore and noted for its royal visitors.

Pass Wynch Bridge and Low Force, and walk upstream for one mile to Holwick Head Bridge. Do not cross the bridge, but climb the hill to enter the Upper Teesdale National Nature Reserve and continue onwards to High Force — surely England's most impressive and finest waterfall. Beyond the waterfall, the path follows the riverside and rounds the bend through juniper bushes and heather to cross three footbridges, erected in 1967, over the Blea, Dry and Skyer Becks. The first footbridge over the Blea Beck with its picturesque waterfall is directly opposite the Dine Holm Quarry, which is an unexpected scene in this wild grandeur. Cross the last footbridge over the Skyer Beck and, in the distance, White Force, on Cronkley Fell, can be seen.

Ascend the Pennine Way through junipers up Bracken Rigg to the black barn at 1,250 feet, then turn north (right) to cross a stepping stile over a wire fence. Walk on past a metal 'Pennine Way' sign by the wall corner, and climb over a tall metal stile to descend below High Crag to a gate in corner of field. Gradually climb up to Cronkley Farm and pass farm buildings on your right ('Pennine Way' sign) to follow farm road and descend to Cronkley Bridge over the Tees. Cross bridge and continue alongside the north

bank of the river for the first time. The path follows Langdon Beck to Saur Hill Bridge (local spelling — Sayer Hill Bridge). Do not cross bridge, but turn right to follow farm road. Pass New House Farm to go through the gate (please shut the gate) and reach the B6277 road. Turn left along road for a few yards to Langdon Beck Youth Hostel on your right.

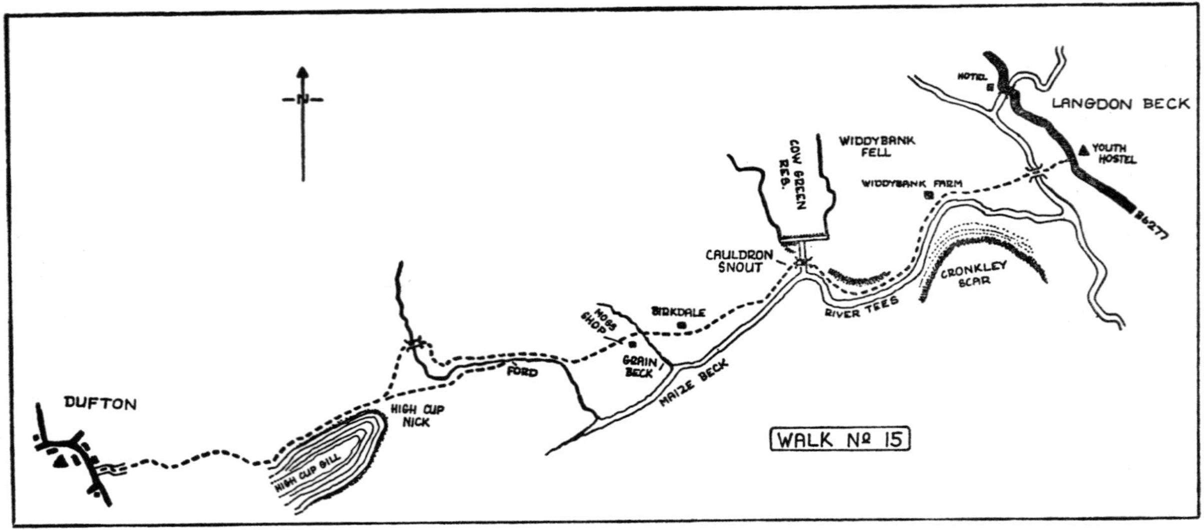

N
LANGDON BECK
HOTEL
YOUTH HOSTEL
B6277
WIDDYBANK FELL
WIDDYBANK FARM
COW GREEN RES.
CAULDRON SNOUT
CRONKLEY SCAR
RIVER TEES
BIRKDALE
MOSS SHOP
GRAIN BECK
MAIZE BECK
FORD
HIGH CUP NICK
HIGH CUP GILL
DUFTON
WALK № 15

15. LANGDON BECK - DUFTON Non-Circular

Route : Langdon Beck - Cauldron Snout - Birkdale - High Cup Nick - Dufton.

Distance : 13½ miles (21.6 kilometres).

Maps : One Inch — Sheets 84, 83. 1:50 000 — Metric Sheets 92, 91. 2½-inch — Sheets NY83, NY82, NY72.

LANGDON BECK HOSTEL, purpose-built, replaced the old hostel which was destroyed by fire in 1958. The hostel is situated close to the Alston-Middleton road and provides excellent views of Upper Teesdale. This final walk is the second longest in the book and should not be attempted in doubtful weather conditions, i.e. fog or snow, because of the rough terrain from Falcon Clints to the Maize Beck.

Leave the hostel, turn left along the B6277 road for a few yards and just before the telephone kiosk and at the Pennine Way sign, turn right through the farm gate (please shut the gate) and walk along the cart road to New House Farm and onwards to Saur (Sayer) Hill Bridge. Cross bridge, walk up track to Saur (Sayer) Hill Farm and take stone stile left of and beyond the farmhouse, to cross a succession of pastures and stone stiles which lead to Widdybank Farm. From the farm, follow Walk 13 in reverse to Cauldron Snout.

Cross the footbridge above the waterfall and follow cart road to Birkdale Farm, reputed to be the loneliest farmstead in England at 1,554 feet above sea level. Two Pennine Way signposts point the way in front of the farm dwellings. Beyond remote Birkdale, the track is onward through two gates and pasture, past another Pennine Way signpost and across Grain Beck. Follow the track over the open moor in a westerly direction veering south-west.

From Grain Beck, climb the moorland track to a big cairn on Moss Shop, former lead mine workings which provide limited shelter. The route ahead is the worst part of the watershed crossing, marked by cairns and posts. It traverses wet peat bog, moorland heather and limestone outcrops, at 1,900 feet above sea level, gradually to descend to the Maize Beck.

My companion and I, on recognisance of this walk, encountered heavy rain and mist for two hours and, despite the defined path, progress was by compass. It is therefore essential to carry a compass and be properly clad.

Follow the Maize Beck to the signpost 'To Footbridge', G.R. 749270, which signifies the flood route along the north bank of the beck to a specially erected footbridge over the beck to High Cup Nick. On this occasion we opted for the flood route from the Maize Beck ford and followed the cairns, also waymarked with black and white posts throughout its length — which are an indicator to divert to the footbridge (care must be taken not to enter the gorge below).

Alternatively, the accepted route is by fording the Maize Beck at this point. (N.B.—The Maize Beck is notoriously dangerous when in flood and has claimed a victim who attempted the crossing). Follow the cairned route along the beckside until it veers away and forward across High Cup plain to the Nick.

From the footbridge, follow cairned route to High Cup Nick, which is an enormous and spectacular ravine resembling a horseshoe, hollowed out of the Pennines. This is the highlight of the walk. Westwards the magnificent views of the Eden Valley and the Lakeland fells can be seen. The path follows the northern edge of the Nick gradually to descend by a cart track to join a metalled lane to the pleasant village of Dufton. The end of the journey and a welcome stay at the newly opened Dufton Youth Hostel can be highly recommended.

ADDITIONAL SUGGESTED WALKS

I list below additional walks for information :—

Part A.

1. Barnard Castle - Marwood - Holme House -Flatts Wood - Barnard Castle. 7 miles.
2. Barnard Castle - Boldron - Kilmond Scar - Startforth - Barnard Castle. 7 miles.
3. Lartington - Butter Stone - Goldsborough - Lartington. 10 miles.
4. Bowes - Gretadale - Brignall Mill - Bowes. 9 miles.
5. Greta Bridge - Brignall Mill - Greta Bridge. 7½ miles.

Part B.

1. Middleton - Coldberry Mine - Aukside - Middleton. 7 miles.
2. Langdon Beck Hotel - Harwood - Langdon Beck Hotel. 10 miles.
3. Langdon Beck Hotel - Dirt Pit - High Force Hotel - Cronkley Bridge - Langdon Beck Hotel. 6½ miles.
4. Holwick - Cronkley Fell - High Force - Holwick. 12 miles.

Part C.

1. Grinton Youth Hostel - Fremington Edge - Hurst - How Tallon - Barningham - Barnard Castle Youth Hostel. 16 miles.
2. Keld Youth Hostel - Tan Hill - Sleightholme - God's Bridge - Bowes - Barnard Castle Youth Hostel. 15 miles.
3. Keld Youth Hostel - Tan Hill - Sleightholme - God's Bridge - Pasture End - Birk Hat - Wythes Hill - Harker Fell - Middleton-in-Teesdale - High Force - Cronkley Bridge - Langdon Beck Youth Hostel. 30 miles.

BIBLIOGRAPHY

The following leaflets and books provide useful background information and interesting further reading :—

Title	Author	Publisher
Walkabout - Barnard Castle	Durham County Council Durham Countryside Officer	Durham County Council
Sidetracks in Teesdale	S. Cardwell	Teesdale Mercury
Upper Teesdale	D. Ramsden	Dalesman Publishing Co.
New Guide to Middleton-in-Teesdale and District	Middeton-in-Teesdale and District Chamber of Trade	Teesdale Mercury
Teesdale	Teesdale Mercury	Teesdale Mercury
Barnard Castle and Teesdale		Barnard Castle Chamber of Trade and Publicity Society
The Pennine Way	K. Oldham	Dalesman Publishing Co.
The Pennine Way	T. Stephenson	H.M.S.O.
The Pennine Way	C. J. Wright	Constable & Co.
Pennine Way Companion	A. Wainwright	Westmorland Gazette Ltd.
Walking in the Northern Dales	The Ramblers' Association	Dalesman Publishing Co.

Portrait of County Durham	P. A. White	Robert Hale
Bowlees Visitor Centre		Durham County Conservation Trust
The Natural History of Upper Teesdale	M. E. Bradshaw	Durham County Conservation Trust

ACKNOWLEDGEMENTS

I would like to thank Dr. T. J. Bines, Nature Conservancy Council; Stan Cardwell, Ramblers' Association, North Yorks and South Durham Area; Simon Hodgson, Durham Countryside Warden; Alan O'Hara, Warden, Barnard Castle Youth Hostel; and M. Salinger, Hon. Secretary, Border and Dales Region, Youth Hostels Association, for their valuable advice. Also, to thank Alan Howe, Michael Leggett, Charles Chapel and Chris Raisbeck, who accompanied me on these Teesdale walks, and especially to thank Mrs. Dorothy Bewick for typing the manuscript.